Hip on Health

Other Redleaf Press Books by Charlotte M. Hendricks

Growing, Growing Strong: A Whole Health Curriculum for Young Children Series (with Connie Jo Smith and Becky S. Bennett)

Body Care

Fitness and Nutrition

Safety

Social and Emotional Well-Being

Community and Environment

Redleaf Quick Guide to Disaster Planning and Preparedness in Early Childhood and School-Age Care Settings (with Michelle Pettibone)

Redleaf Quick Guide to Medical Emergencies in Early Childhood Settings

Hip *on* HEALTH

Health Information for Caregivers and Families

CHARLOTTE M. HENDRICKS, PhD

Illustrations by Nic Frising

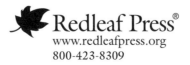

Redleaf Press®
www.redleafpress.org
800-423-8309

To Kevin, who started this, and to Nikki.

Published by Redleaf Press
10 Yorkton Court
St. Paul, MN 55117
www.redleafpress.org

First edition 2015
Cover design by Ryan Scheife, Mayfly Design
Cover illustrations by Nic Frising
Interior illustrations by Nic Frising
Printed in the United States of America
21 20 19 18 17 16 15 14   1 2 3 4 5 6 7 8

Library of Congress Cataloging-in-Publication Data
Hendricks, Charlotte Mitchell, 1957-
  Hip on health : health information for caregivers and families /
Charlotte Hendricks ; illustrations by Nic Frising. — First edition.
     pages cm
  ISBN 978-1-60554-401-4 (pbk. : alk. paper)
1. Health--Popular works. 2. Medicine, Preventive. 3. Self-care,
Health—Popular works. I. Title.
  RA776.H516 2015
  613—dc23
                              2014023042

Printed on acid-free paper

Contents

Dear Reader,

Do you have questions about common childhood illnesses? Do you want easy-to-read information on preventing injuries? Are you looking for ways to share important health and safety topics with parents, families, and caregivers?

If so, then *Hip on Health* is for you!

This practical resource was developed to help parents, families, teachers, and caregivers learn more about keeping young children healthy and safe. *Hip on Health* contains information you can easily distribute on 143 different topics related to children's growth and development, childhood illnesses, health care and illness prevention, infant care, nutrition, indoor and outdoor safety, and social-emotional behavior. Each topic in *Hip on Health* comes in two reproducible forms:

✓ An 8.5 x 11-inch miniposter that you can photocopy and display.

The miniposters include clear, concise content and appealing graphics to attract attention and increase awareness of important children's health, safety, and development topics. Display the miniposters at the front desk, in the classroom, on a family-information bulletin board, in the break room, and near the main entrance—wherever they're likely to catch attention. And with 143 different topics, you can post different miniposters each week. (There's room saved at the bottom of each miniposter to include your organization's logo, if you'd like to personalize the information.)

✓ An 8.5 x 11-inch information sheet that you can photocopy and distribute.

The information sheets provide more detail related to the content in the miniposters. Each information sheet includes a fun cartoon strip and three or four facts related to the topic, along with specific recommendations for actions to promote children's health, safety, and development. You can photocopy these easy-to-read sheets and send them home with the children, include them in newsletters, and distribute them at parent and staff meetings to support conversations and training opportunities.

Children depend on adults to keep them healthy and safe. *Hip on Health* provides important and accurate health and safety information—information that has been researched and widely field-tested—in an engaging way that families and caregivers will remember.

With thanks for the work you do to promote children's health,

Charlotte M. Hendricks

Chicken Pox

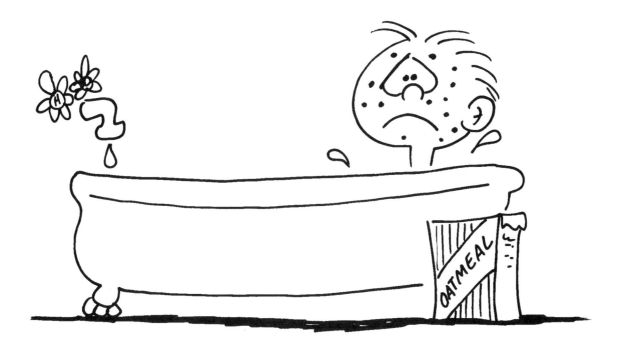

Chicken pox can be prevented by immunization.

The chicken pox virus is very contagious. A child with chicken pox should stay away from other children until all the spots have crusted over and dried. This takes about one week.

Cut the child's fingernails short to prevent scratching. Baths with oatmeal may reduce the itching. Ask the child's doctor about medicine to reduce fever and itching.

From *Hip on Health: Health Information for Caregivers and Families* by Charlotte M. Hendricks. Published by Redleaf Press. www.redleafpress.org.

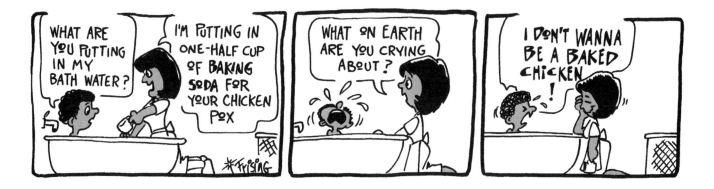

Chicken Pox

Chicken pox is a rash caused by a virus. The rash forms small bumps that turn into blisters. The sores also can affect internal organs and cause serious complications. Other symptoms of chicken pox include tiredness, fever, and headache.

The rash may itch. Cut the child's fingernails very short to prevent scratching. Scratching the blisters can cause further infection and scarring.

Warm baths with oatmeal or baking soda may reduce the itching. Here is how to prepare these treatments:

✓ Place 1 cup of plain uncooked oatmeal in a stocking or net bag. Swish it through the warm bath water.

✓ Put ½ cup of baking soda in a tub of warm water.

Ask the child's doctor about medication to reduce fever or itching.

✓ Do not give aspirin to children! Aspirin has been associated with the development of Reye syndrome, a rare but life-threatening condition.

✓ Do not use hydrocortisone or antihistamine creams and sprays.

Chicken pox spreads easily among children, even before the rash appears. A child with chicken pox should stay away from other children until all the spots have crusted over and dried. This usually takes about one week.

Chicken pox can be prevented through immunization. This immunization is usually given when the child is twelve to fifteen months old. This vaccine not only prevents chicken pox; it also helps prevent shingles later in life. Shingles is a skin rash caused by the same virus that causes chicken pox.

From *Hip on Health: Health Information for Caregivers and Families* by Charlotte M. Hendricks. Published by Redleaf Press. www.redleafpress.org.

Diphtheria

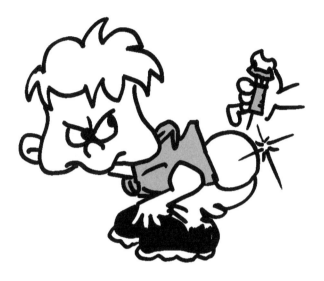

Diphtheria causes a sore throat, slight fever, and chills. Sometimes a thick membrane forms across children's throats, making it hard to swallow or breathe. About 10 percent of people who get diphtheria die from it.

Diphtheria is preventable. All children should be immunized against diphtheria.

From *Hip on Health: Health Information for Caregivers and Families* by Charlotte M. Hendricks. Published by Redleaf Press. www.redleafpress.org.

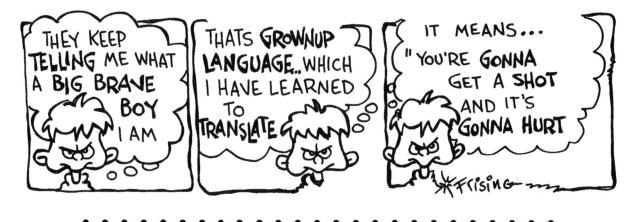

Diphtheria

Diphtheria is caused by bacteria that live in the mouth, throat, and nose of infected people. It is easily spread through coughing or sneezing.

Diphtheria usually causes a sore throat, slight fever, and chills. If the disease is not diagnosed and treated early, it can produce a powerful toxin (poison) that spreads throughout the body. This can cause serious complications such as heart failure, suffocation, paralysis, and death.

Sometimes a thick membrane forms across children's throats, making it hard to swallow or breathe. Approximately 10 percent of people who get diphtheria die from it; the death rate is even higher among young children.

Diphtheria is preventable through immunization. Diphtheria once was a major cause of childhood illness and death. Because of immunizations, diphtheria is very rare in the United States. However, the disease still exists in other countries.

All children should be immunized! The diphtheria vaccine is part of the DTaP injection. It usually is given to children at two months, four months, and six months of age. A booster is given at fifteen to eighteen months and again at four to six years. Another booster, the Tdap injection, is given at eleven to twelve years of age.

From *Hip on Health: Health Information for Caregivers and Families* by Charlotte M. Hendricks. Published by Redleaf Press. www.redleafpress.org.

Hepatitis

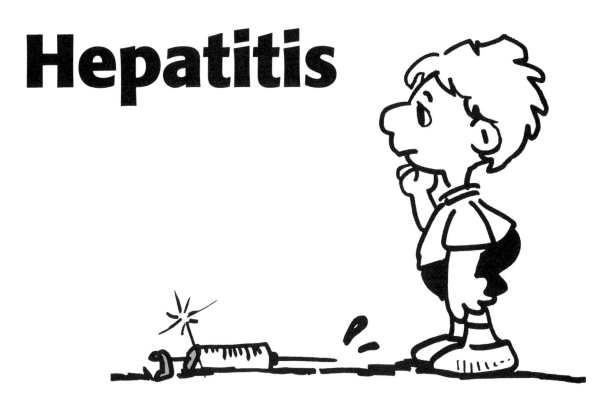

Hepatitis is a viral disease that causes inflammation of the liver. It can be deadly. Hepatitis A is spread through contaminated food and drink. Hepatitis B can be spread through infected blood and blood products.

Children can get hepatitis by touching the blood of someone who is already infected. They can also become infected if they stick or cut themselves with a contaminated object, such as a needle or razor. Teach children to avoid touching blood and objects that may have blood on them.

Protect children and yourself by getting immunized against hepatitis A and hepatitis B.

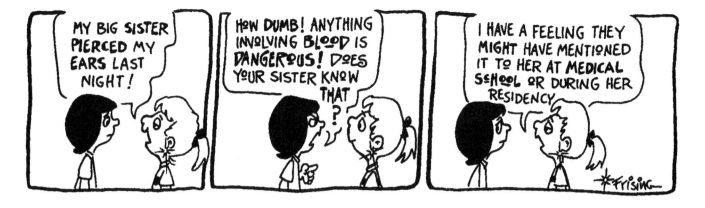

Hepatitis

Hepatitis is a disease that causes inflammation of the liver. This disease can be deadly. There are several types of hepatitis. Each is caused by a different virus and is spread, treated, and prevented differently.

Hepatitis A can be spread when someone who is infected does not wash hands properly after using the toilet. It is also found in sewage. You can get hepatitis A by eating raw oysters and shellfish from water contaminated by sewage.

Hepatitis B is spread through infected blood and blood products. Children can also be infected if they stick or cut themselves with a contaminated object, such as a needle or razor.

Teach children to avoid touching blood and objects that may have blood on them.

Hepatitis C is also spread through infected blood. In past years, it was usually spread by blood transfusions, but the blood supply in the United States is now screened and treated to be safe for transfusions.

The number of people with hepatitis is increasing. You can help protect children and yourself by getting immunized against hepatitis A and hepatitis B. Doctors often give the first shot to newborn infants before they leave the hospital. Be sure children have all the recommended immunizations.

From *Hip on Health: Health Information for Caregivers and Families* by Charlotte M. Hendricks. Published by Redleaf Press. www.redleafpress.org.

Hib

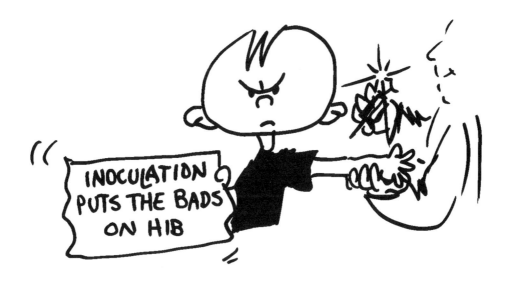

Hib (*Haemophilus influenzae* type b) is an airborne bacterial disease. It is spread by coughing, sneezing, and talking.

Hib can cause serious complications in young children, such as ear infections, meningitis, pneumonia, deafness, seizures, and intellectual disability.

Hib is preventable. All children under the age of 5 should be immunized against Hib.

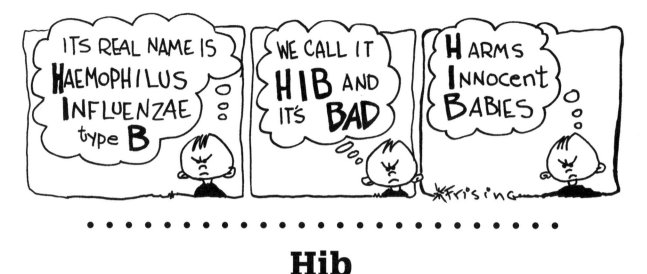

ITS REAL NAME IS **HAEMOPHILUS INFLUENZAE** type **B**

WE CALL IT **HIB** AND IT'S **BAD**

HARMS **I**NNOCENT **B**ABIES

Hib

Hib (*Haemophilus influenzae* type b) is a bacterial disease spread through the air by coughing, sneezing, and talking.

Hib bacteria enter children's noses or throats. If they stay there, the children probably will not become sick. But sometimes the bacteria spread to the lungs or bloodstream, causing serious complications including ear infection, meningitis, and pneumonia.

Hib can also cause epiglottitis, an inflammation and swelling in the throat that can make it hard to breathe. Hib also can cause deafness, seizures, and intellectual disability.

This disease is most dangerous for children younger than five years, especially infants.

Hib is preventable. All children younger than five years should be immunized. They should get the vaccine at two and four months and, depending on the brand of vaccine given, possibly another dose at six months. Children need a booster dose between twelve and fifteen months.

HIV and AIDS

The human immunodeficiency virus (HIV) can lead to acquired immunodeficiency syndrome (AIDS). HIV is spread by blood and body fluids from an infected individual.

Teach children about diseases, and specifically these facts about HIV and AIDS:

- Blood can contain germs that make you sick. Never touch anyone else's blood.

- You cannot get HIV/AIDS from hugging or touching someone's hand.

- You cannot get HIV/AIDS from playing tag, hide-and-seek, or coloring pictures with someone.

From *Hip on Health: Health Information for Caregivers and Families* by Charlotte M. Hendricks. Published by Redleaf Press. www.redleafpress.org.

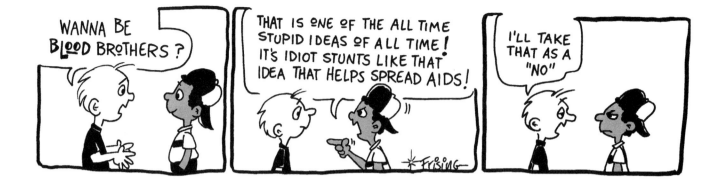

HIV and AIDS

The human immunodeficiency virus (HIV) can lead to acquired immunodeficiency syndrome (AIDS). HIV is spread by blood and body fluids from an infected individual. A person who has been infected with the virus is "HIV positive." They may have no symptoms, but can transmit the virus to others.

HIV destroys the body's immune system so the body cannot fight diseases. There is no vaccine to prevent HIV infection.

HIV and AIDS are *not* common in young children. Most children with HIV infection were infected during or before birth by mothers with HIV infection. Children can get the disease, however, by touching blood or body fluids from an infected person. Here are some concepts you can teach children about infectious diseases, and specifically about HIV and AIDS:

✓ Blood can contain germs that make you sick. Never touch or taste anyone else's blood.

✓ Do not touch objects that may have blood on them, such as needles or weapons.

✓ You cannot get HIV or AIDS from being in the same room with someone who has it. You cannot get HIV/AIDS from hugging or touching someone's hand.

✓ If another child is HIV positive, it is okay for children to play with him or her. Children cannot get HIV/AIDS from playing tag, hide-and-seek, or coloring pictures with a child infected with HIV or a child with AIDS.

From *Hip on Health: Health Information for Caregivers and Families* by Charlotte M. Hendricks. Published by Redleaf Press. www.redleafpress.org.

Influenza

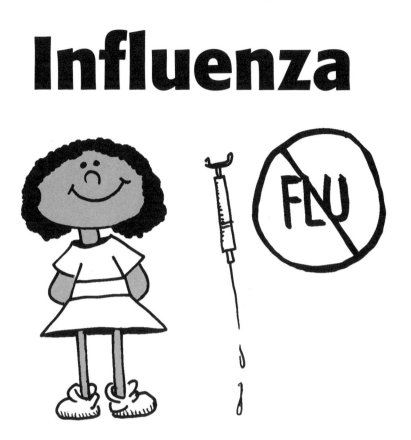

Influenza (the flu) is a viral disease that causes fever, cough, sore throat, runny or stuffy nose, headache, muscle ache, and fatigue.

Yearly flu vaccinations are recommended for all children 6 months of age and older and for all adults.

Flu vaccine can be given in two ways. The flu shot is given with a needle, usually in the arm. It is recommended for children over 6 months of age.

Healthy children over age 2 may be given a nasal-spray flu vaccine instead.

From *Hip on Health: Health Information for Caregivers and Families* by Charlotte M. Hendricks. Published by Redleaf Press. www.redleafpress.org.

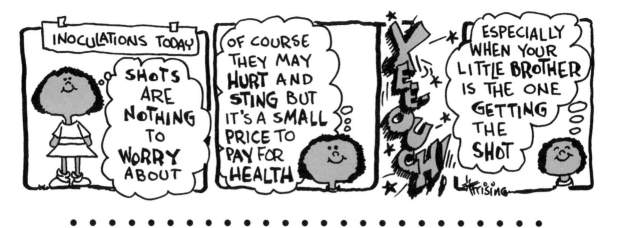

Influenza

Influenza (flu) is a viral infection that causes fever, cough, sore throat, runny or stuffy nose, headache, muscle ache, and fatigue. A child's doctor may recommend an over-the-counter medication to reduce fever and discomfort. Never give aspirin to children with viral illnesses like the flu! Aspirin has been associated with the development of Reye syndrome, a rare but life-threatening condition.

Most people who get the flu recover fully within one to two weeks. However, some people develop serious complications, such as pneumonia.

The annual flu season is usually from November through April. During this time, flu viruses circulate widely. An annual flu vaccination is the best way to reduce the chance of getting the flu.

Yearly flu vaccinations are recommended for children six months of age and older and for all adults.

Flu vaccine can be given in two ways. The flu shot, usually given in the arm, is approved for use among people six months of age or older, including healthy people and those with chronic medical conditions.

A different kind of vaccine can be given in a nasal (nose) spray. It is approved for use among healthy people two to forty-nine years of age.

The flu virus changes, so the vaccine is different each year. The vaccine protects against the influenza virus strains expected for that year.

From *Hip on Health: Health Information for Caregivers and Families* by Charlotte M. Hendricks. Published by Redleaf Press. www.redleafpress.org.

Measles

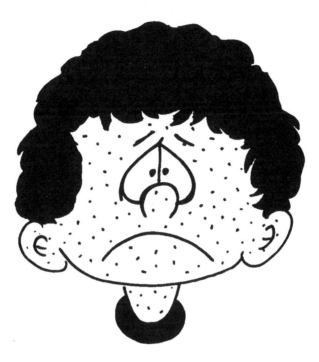

Measles is a serious viral disease.

Measles is easily spread through the air. Children can get measles from infected people who cough or sneeze around them, talk to them, or are simply in the same room with them.

Measles is preventable. All children should be immunized against measles. The vaccine is usually given as part of the measles, mumps, and rubella (MMR) immunization. The first dose is given at 12 to 15 months. The second dose is usually given at 4 to 6 years.

From *Hip on Health: Health Information for Caregivers and Families* by Charlotte M. Hendricks. Published by Redleaf Press. www.redleafpress.org.

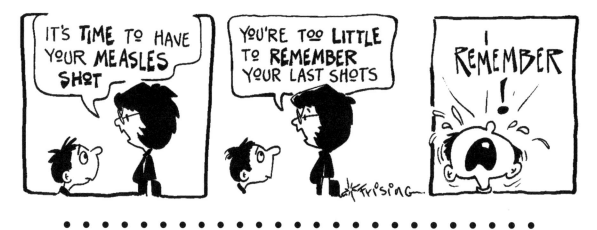

Measles

Measles is a very contagious viral disease that spreads easily through the air. Children can get measles from infected people who cough or sneeze around them, talk to them, or are in the same room with them.

Measles begins with a fever that lasts for a couple of days, followed by a cough, runny nose, and conjunctivitis (pinkeye). A rash starts on the face and upper neck, spreads down the back and trunk, then extends to the arms, hands, legs, and feet. After about five days, the rash fades in the same order it appeared.

A child's doctor may recommend an over-the-counter medication to reduce fever and discomfort. Never give aspirin to children with viral illnesses like measles! Aspirin has been associated with the development of Reye syndrome, a rare but life-threatening condition.

Measles can have serious complications, such as diarrhea, ear infection, croup, pneumonia, and encephalitis. Encephalitis, an inflammation of the brain, can cause deafness, intellectual disability, and death.

Measles is preventable! All children should be immunized. Measles is not common in the United States because most children are immunized. However, the disease is common in other countries and can easily be brought into the United States.

The measles vaccine is usually given as part of the measles, mumps, and rubella (MMR) immunization. The first dose is given at twelve to fifteen months. The second dose is usually given at four to six years.

From *Hip on Health: Health Information for Caregivers and Families* by Charlotte M. Hendricks. Published by Redleaf Press. www.redleafpress.org.

Meningitis

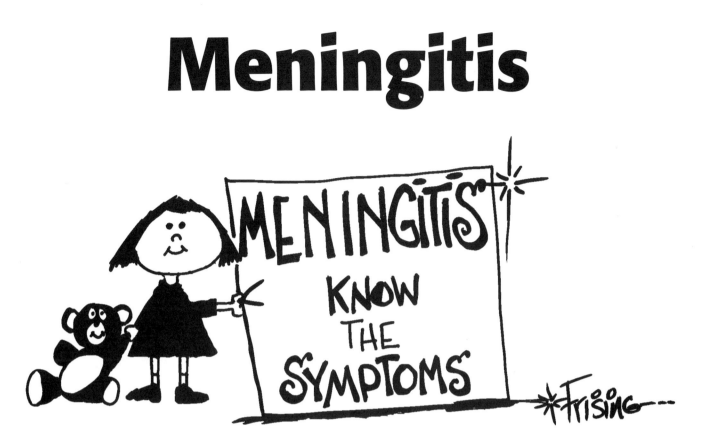

Meningitis is a rare disease, and it can be very serious. Meningitis is an inflammation of the membranes and fluid surrounding the brain and spinal cord.

The disease may be mild, causing headache and fever. It can also be severe and even life threatening.

Diseases such as chicken pox, mumps, and Hib can lead to meningitis. Make sure children have all recommended immunizations.

From *Hip on Health: Health Information for Caregivers and Families* by Charlotte M. Hendricks. Published by Redleaf Press. www.redleafpress.org.

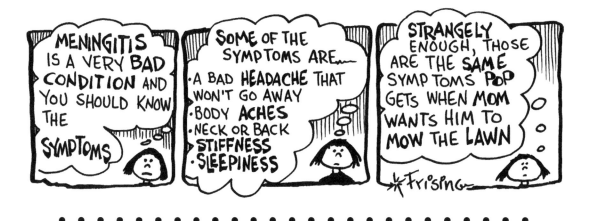

Meningitis

Meningitis is a rare disease, and it can be very serious. It is an inflammation of the membranes and fluid surrounding the brain and spinal cord. It is sometimes called spinal meningitis.

Call the child's doctor if you notice these symptoms:

✓ high fever

✓ headache

✓ neck stiffness or back stiffness

✓ eye pain or irritation when exposed to light

✓ nausea or vomiting, body aches, and fever

✓ sleepiness or confusion

In infants, the only symptoms may be slowness or inactivity, irritability, vomiting, or poor feeding. Trust your intuition. If you think an infant is sick, call the infant's doctor.

Meningitis can be treated, but the best treatment is prevention! It is usually caused by viral or bacterial infections, such as measles, chicken pox, mumps, pneumococcal disease, and Hib. These and some other diseases can be prevented by immunizations. Make sure children are up to date on recommended immunizations.

A vaccine to prevent meningococcal infection, a more common cause of meningitis in teenagers and young adults, is available and recommended for children once they reach eleven to twelve years. Vaccination is also recommended for children and adults with specific risks. Ask a doctor for recommendations for you or other family members.

From *Hip on Health: Health Information for Caregivers and Families* by Charlotte M. Hendricks. Published by Redleaf Press. www.redleafpress.org.

Mumps

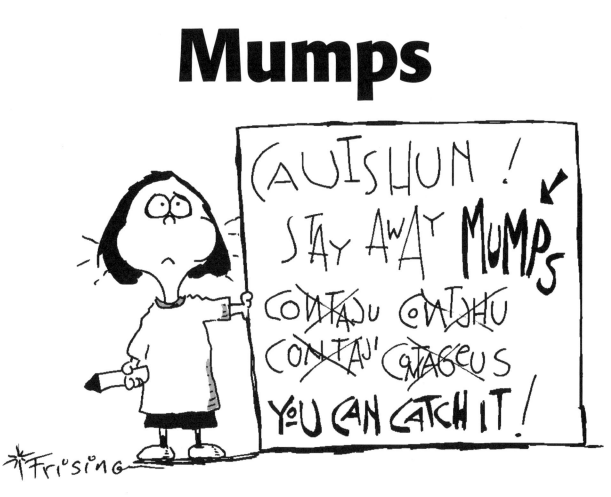

Mumps is a viral disease that can cause fever, muscle ache, and pain and swelling of the cheeks and jaw.

Mumps is usually a mild disease. However, it can have serious complications.

All children should be immunized against mumps. The vaccine is usually given as part of the measles, mumps, and rubella (MMR) immunization. The first dose is given at 12 to 15 months. The second dose is usually given at 4 to 6 years.

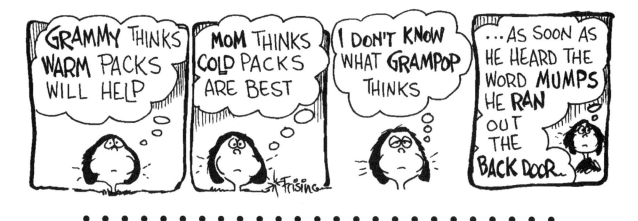

Mumps

Mumps is caused by a virus. It is spread through the air by coughing, sneezing, or talking.

Mumps is usually mild and lasts about ten days. It can cause fever, headache, muscle ache, tiredness, and pain and swelling of the cheeks and jaw because of inflammation in the salivary glands. This pain becomes worse when infected children swallow, talk, chew, or drink juice that is acidic (such as orange juice).

The most common complication of mumps is inflammation of the testicles in teenage or adult men. Mumps can lead to more serious complications, including meningitis (inflammation of the covering of the brain and spinal cord), encephalitis (inflammation of the brain), and deafness.

Mumps is preventable, and all children should be immunized. The vaccine is usually given as part of the measles, mumps, and rubella (MMR) immunization. The first dose is given at twelve to fifteen months. The second dose is usually given at four to six years.

If you think a child has mumps, call the child's doctor immediately.

Never give aspirin to children who have viral illnesses like mumps. Aspirin has been associated with the development of Reye syndrome, a rare but life-threatening condition.

From *Hip on Health: Health Information for Caregivers and Families* by Charlotte M. Hendricks. Published by Redleaf Press. www.redleafpress.org.

Pertussis

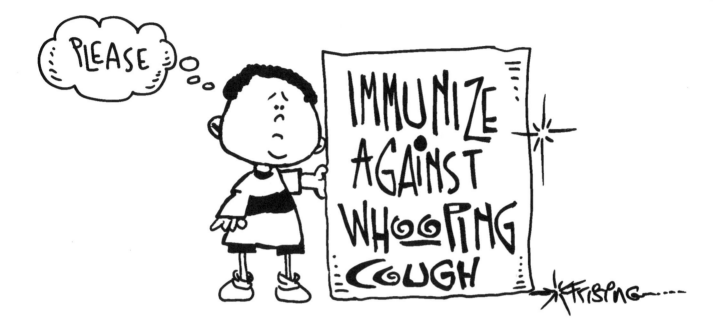

Pertussis (whooping cough) is a bacterial infection of the respiratory system. It causes severe coughing spells that can last for weeks. Between coughing spells, children may gasp for air with whooping sounds.

The coughing and vomiting associated with pertussis make it difficult for children to drink, eat, and breathe. The disease is most serious in infants and young children.

Pertussis is preventable. All children should be immunized against pertussis. The vaccine is part of the DTaP injection.

From *Hip on Health: Health Information for Caregivers and Families* by Charlotte M. Hendricks. Published by Redleaf Press. www.redleafpress.org.

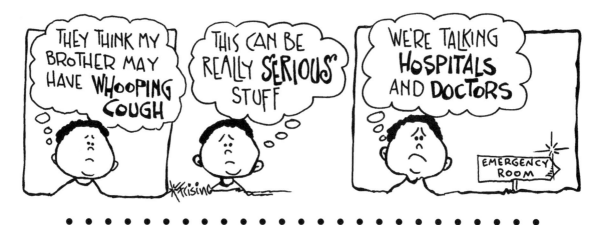

Pertussis

Pertussis (whooping cough) is a bacterial infection of the respiratory system. Children cough violently and rapidly, over and over, until they have expelled the air from their lungs. Then they inhale with loud whooping sounds. The coughing begins again. Whooping cough can continue for several weeks.

Severe coughing can cause children to turn blue in the face or vomit. Coughing and vomiting can make it difficult for children to drink, eat, and breathe.

The disease is most serious in infants and young children. Infants may stop breathing for a few seconds. Infants and young children with pertussis often need hospital treatment.

Pertussis can lead to other complications, such as pneumonia, and to death.

Pertussis is caused by bacteria and is easily spread through coughing or sneezing. But it is preventable.

All children should be immunized. The vaccine is part of the DTaP injection. It is usually given to children at two, four, and six months of age, with boosters at fifteen to eighteen months, and again at four to six years. Another booster, the Tdap injection, is given at eleven to twelve years of age.

Pneumococcal Disease

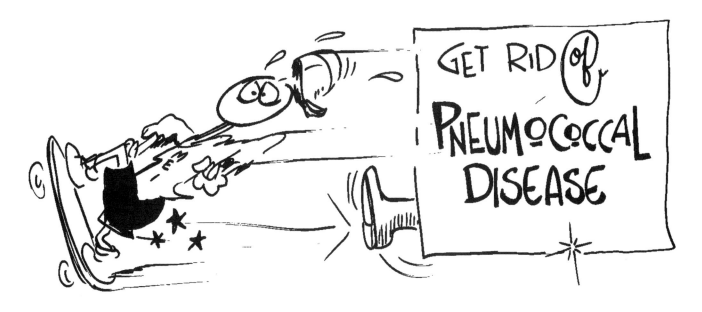

The *Streptococcus pneumoniae*, a bacterium, is a leading cause of middle ear infections in children. It can also cause pneumonia, sinus infection, and meningitis.

Many cases of pneumococcal disease are preventable through immunization.

Immunization requires four doses of the vaccine—one dose at 2, 4, and 6 months and a booster dose at 12 to 15 months.

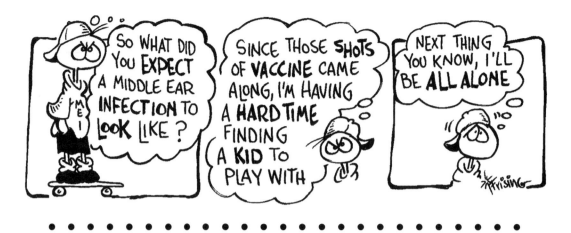

Pneumococcal Disease

Streptococcus pneumococcus is a leading cause of middle ear infections in children, as well as pneumonia, sinus infection, and meningitis.

Children under two years, children in group child care, and children with certain chronic illnesses are at higher risk for pneumococcal disease. The bacteria are spread through coughing and sneezing. People, especially children, may carry the bacteria in their throats without being ill from it, and they can spread it.

Pneumococcal disease can be very serious in young children, causing ear infections, meningitis, bacteremia (bacteria in the blood), and other invasive diseases. Young children die each year from pneumococcal infection.

Pneumococcal disease is treated with antibiotics, although the bacteria are becoming more resistant to penicillin and other antibiotic treatments.

Many cases of pneumococcal disease are preventable through immunization. The vaccine is very effective in preventing pneumococcal disease in young children, including most meningitis infections and many ear infections.

All children should be immunized. Immunization requires four doses of the vaccine—one at two, four, and six months, and a booster at twelve to fifteen months.

From *Hip on Health: Health Information for Caregivers and Families* by Charlotte M. Hendricks. Published by Redleaf Press. www.redleafpress.org.

Polio

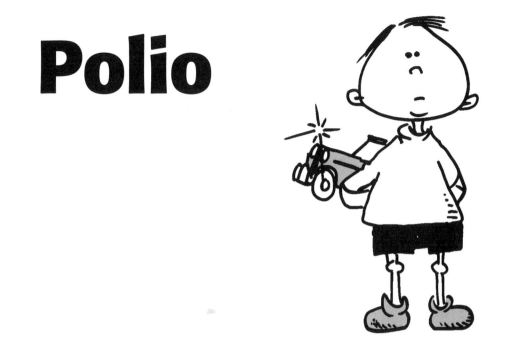

Polio is a viral disease that can cause paralysis and other serious problems. There is no polio in the United States now, thanks to immunization, but the disease still exists in other parts of the world. It would take only one person with polio traveling from another country to bring the disease here to people who are not protected by vaccines.

Sometimes polio is a mild illness, much like a cold. But sometimes it causes paralysis. There is no antibiotic available to treat polio.

Polio is preventable. All children should be immunized against polio.

From *Hip on Health: Health Information for Caregivers and Families* by Charlotte M. Hendricks. Published by Redleaf Press. www.redleafpress.org.

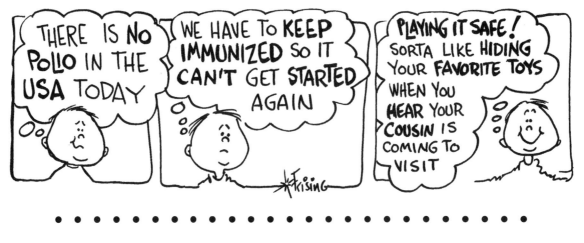

Polio

Polio is a viral disease spread through contact with the bowel movements of infected persons (for instance, by changing diapers) and through coughing, sneezing, and contaminated mucus.

Sometimes it is mild, much like a cold. Severe illness affects the muscles and can cause paralysis. It usually affects the child's legs. Sometimes polio affects other muscles, including those that control breathing. There is no antibiotic treatment for polio, and children can die from it.

The polio vaccine became widely used in the 1950s. Before then, the disease caused thousands of cases of paralysis and other serious disorders every year. There are no cases of polio in the United States now, thanks to immunization. However, the disease still exists in some parts of the world. It would take only one case of polio from another country to bring the disease back if we are not protected by vaccine.

Polio is preventable! All children should be immunized. The polio vaccine (IPV) shot used in the United States contains killed virus.

Children should get a polio shot at two, four, and six to eighteen months, and at four to six years.

From *Hip on Health: Health Information for Caregivers and Families* by Charlotte M. Hendricks. Published by Redleaf Press. www.redleafpress.org.

RSV

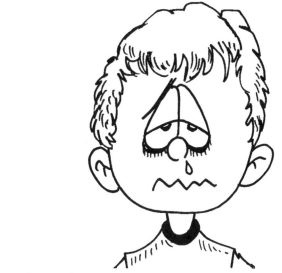

Respiratory syncytial virus (RSV) is a common virus that can cause respiratory illness in young children. It usually mimics a common cold, causing runny nose and mild cough. But RSV infection can lead to serious complications. Call a doctor if children have any of these symptoms:

- fever in infants under three months, or temperature above 100°F in older infants

- fever along with listlessness, confusion, irritability, neck stiffness, or other symptoms

- trouble breathing

- thick nasal discharge, worsening cough, or coughing up mucus

RSV is very contagious. The best way to prevent RSV infection is to wash hands often.

From *Hip on Health: Health Information for Caregivers and Families* by Charlotte M. Hendricks. Published by Redleaf Press. www.redleafpress.org.

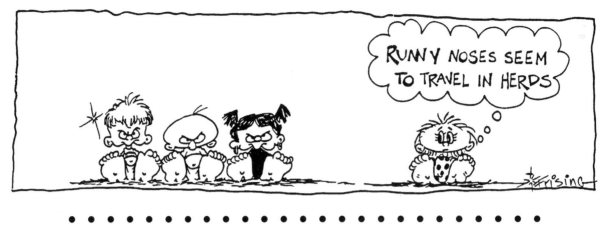

RSV

Respiratory syncytial virus (RSV) is a common, highly contagious virus that causes respiratory illness in young children. Many young children in child care and other group settings contract RSV. The disease is most common during late fall through early spring.

Symptoms of RSV usually mimic those of the common cold, such as a runny nose and mild cough. Over the next few days, the symptoms worsen, and children may develop hacking coughs, high fevers, wheezing, and difficulty breathing. Most children recover within one to two weeks, but they can get RSV again.

This disease can be more serious in infants, young children, and children who have other chronic illnesses. It can lead to serious complications, such as bronchial infections and pneumonia.

Call a doctor if children have any of these symptoms:

✓ fever in infants under three months or temperatures above 100°F in older infants

✓ fever along with listlessness, confusion, irritability, neck stiffness, or other symptoms

✓ trouble breathing

✓ thick nasal discharge

✓ cough that worsens or coughing up mucus

The infection is contagious and can be passed on by people with no symptoms of RSV. It is easily spread by sneezing or coughing and can be transmitted by hands, clothing, used tissues, and surfaces, such as toys and tables.

The best way to prevent RSV and other illness is to wash hands often with soap and running water.

Teach children to cough and sneeze into their elbows. Help them learn to use tissues to cover their sneezes and coughs. Dispose of used tissues, and tell them to wash their hands again!

Rubella

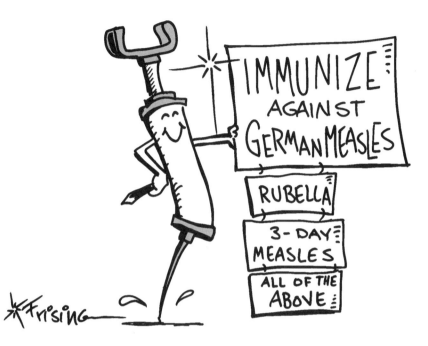

Rubella is sometimes called German measles or three-day measles. It causes mild fever and swollen glands in the neck or behind the ears. A rash appears but does not itch.

Rubella is preventable, and all children should be immunized against rubella. The vaccine is usually given as part of the measles, mumps, and rubella (MMR) immunization.

The greatest danger from rubella is to unborn infants. Women should ask their doctor about receiving rubella vaccine before they become pregnant.

From *Hip on Health: Health Information for Caregivers and Families* by Charlotte M. Hendricks. Published by Redleaf Press. www.redleafpress.org.

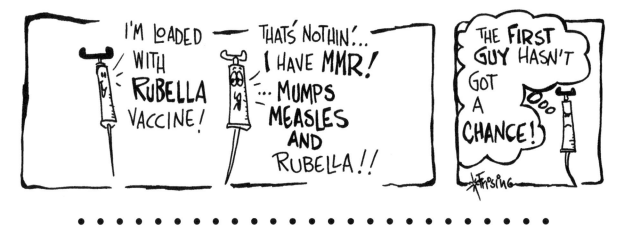

Rubella

Rubella is sometimes called German or three-day measles. It is rare in the United States because of immunization. However, outbreaks continue to occur in groups of unimmunized people.

Rubella is usually mild in children. It begins with slight fever and swollen glands in the neck or behind the ears. On the second or third day, a rash appears at the hairline and spreads downward over the rest of the body. The rash does not itch and lasts three to five days.

When an unvaccinated pregnant woman contracts rubella in the early months of her pregnancy, the chance that her child will be born with birth defects is high. Rubella can cause premature delivery, miscarriage, stillbirth, and serious birth defects, such as heart abnormalities, intellectual disability, blindness, and deafness. Women should be tested for immunity and ask their doctor about the rubella vaccine before they become pregnant.

Call a doctor if you think children have rubella. Never give aspirin to children with viral illnesses like rubella! Aspirin has been associated with the development of Reye syndrome, a rare but life-threatening condition.

Rubella is preventable, and all children should be immunized against rubella. The vaccine is usually given as part of the measles, mumps, and rubella (MMR) immunization. The first dose is given at twelve to fifteen months. The second dose is usually given at four to six years.

From *Hip on Health: Health Information for Caregivers and Families* by Charlotte M. Hendricks. Published by Redleaf Press. www.redleafpress.org.

Tetanus

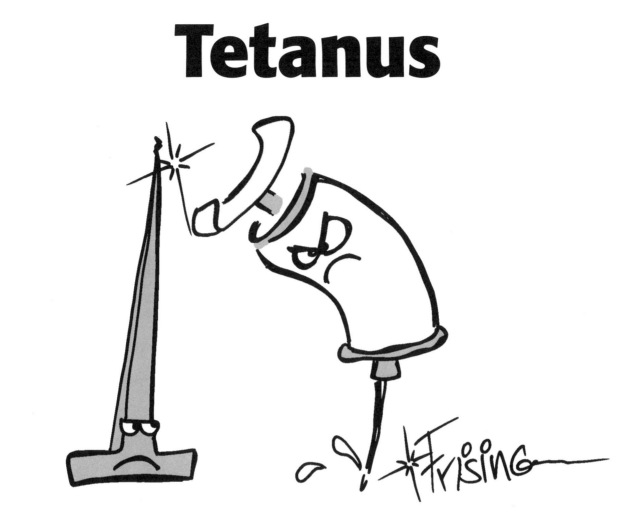

Tetanus is a rare but serious disease caused when the tetanus bacteria enter a cut, scratch, bite, or other wound. Tetanus affects the muscles and nerves. Tetanus can be fatal.

Tetanus is preventable. Children (and adults) should receive immunizations to prevent this disease. Tetanus is the *T* in the DTaP series of injections.

Adults should receive tetanus boosters every 10 years.

From *Hip on Health: Health Information for Caregivers and Families* by Charlotte M. Hendricks. Published by Redleaf Press. www.redleafpress.org.

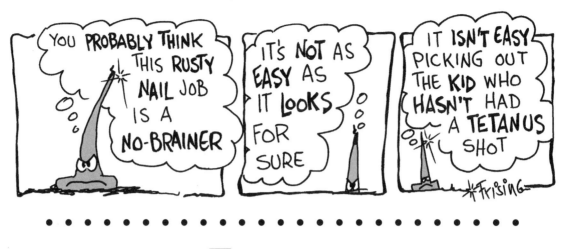

Tetanus

Tetanus—which is sometimes called lockjaw—is a rare but serious disease of the nervous system. The disease occurs when tetanus bacteria get into deep puncture wounds and create a toxin.

Tetanus affects the muscles and nerves. It often begins with muscle spasms in the jaw, difficulty in swallowing, and stiffness or pain in the muscles of the neck, shoulder, or back. Muscle spasms soon spread to the abdomen, upper arms, and thighs. Tetanus can be treated if diagnosed early, but it is still a very serious disease.

Many people think rusty nails cause tetanus, but it is the bacteria, not the rust. Children can get tetanus from shiny nails just as easily.

Any type of wound can become infected—a puncture wound, cut, scratch, burn, or animal bite. Injuries can be so small that you may not notice them. Always clean children's wounds thoroughly. However, cleaning wounds is not a substitute for immunization.

Tetanus is preventable. All children (and adults) should be immunized. The vaccine is part of the DTaP injection. It is usually given to children at two, four, and six months. A booster is given at fifteen to eighteen months and again at four to six years. Another booster, the Tdap injection, is given at eleven to twelve years of age.

Adults should have tetanus boosters every ten years. Tetanus boosters may also be given after injuries.

From *Hip on Health: Health Information for Caregivers and Families* by Charlotte M. Hendricks. Published by Redleaf Press. www.redleafpress.org.

Tuberculosis

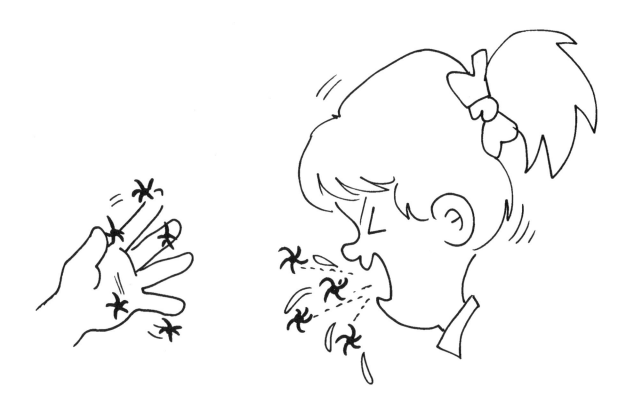

Tuberculosis (TB) is a respiratory disease caused by bacteria. It is spread from person to person through the air. Children can be exposed to TB through close contact with anyone who has the disease.

If you think children have been exposed to TB, ask a doctor or the health department about a TB skin test or blood test.

Tuberculosis usually can be cured when treated early.

From *Hip on Health: Health Information for Caregivers and Families* by Charlotte M. Hendricks. Published by Redleaf Press. www.redleafpress.org.

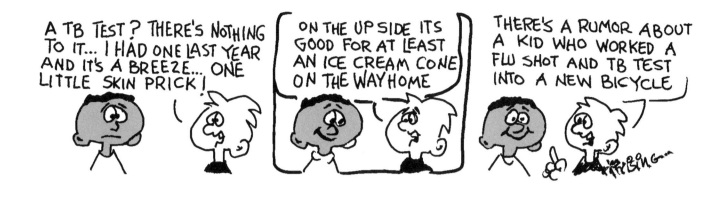

Tuberculosis

Tuberculosis (TB) is a disease caused by bacteria. It is spread from person to person through the air.

When the bacteria enter the body, the disease develops slowly. Infected people may not have any symptoms for years. But if the infection becomes active, it usually affects the lungs. It can affect other parts of the body, including the bones, kidneys, and brain. It can cause chronic illness and death if not treated.

Children can be exposed to TB through close contact with someone who has the disease. If you think children have been exposed to TB, call their doctors or the health department about a TB skin test or a blood test.

The skin test is a tiny skin prick. In two days, take children back to the clinic so a nurse can look at the spot. If the spots are red and swollen, it means the children have been exposed to TB. It does not mean they have an active case of the disease.

When children have been exposed, their doctors may prescribe a medicine that helps prevent the disease. Tuberculosis usually can be cured if treated early.

From *Hip on Health: Health Information for Caregivers and Families* by Charlotte M. Hendricks. Published by Redleaf Press. www.redleafpress.org.

Authorization

Child caregivers must know names of individuals trusted to pick up each child. The child care program should check picture identification.

Parents should provide current home, work, and cell phone numbers.

From *Hip on Health: Health Information for Caregivers and Families* by Charlotte M. Hendricks. Published by Redleaf Press. www.redleafpress.org.

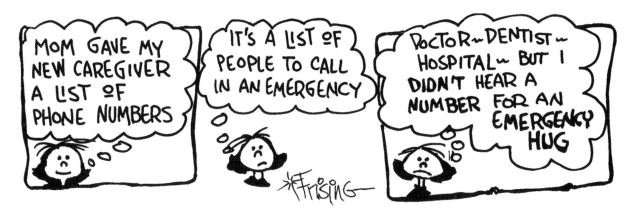

Authorization

Child caregivers want to give the best care possible to each child. Parents can help by providing information and written authorizations to caregivers.

The parents or guardians may not always be the person who picks up a child. Caregivers need to know the names of trusted individuals to pick up each child and should check picture identification. Emergency situations may require that a person not on the authorization list pick up a child. Caregivers should let parents know how they will handle such situations.

It is also important for caregivers to know if there are certain persons who must never pick up a child. For example, if parental custody is an issue, then the custodial parent should give the caregiver legal documentation specifying who may pick up or visit the child.

Children's caregivers should also have the following information:

✓ current phone numbers (home, work, and cell) for parents and others who can pick up children

✓ authorization to seek medical treatment for children when needed

✓ name and telephone number for child's doctor, preferred hospital or clinic, and insurance information

Buckle Up

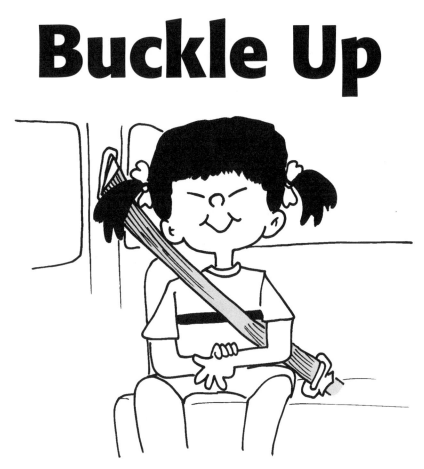

Motor vehicle accidents are a leading cause of injury and death among young children. A crash at just 5 miles per hour can throw an unbuckled child into the dashboard or windshield.

Infants and small children should use safety seats (car seats). Older children should use booster seats along with lap belts and shoulder harness.

Children are more likely to buckle themselves up if they see you buckle up too. Teach them to always buckle up and ride the safe way.

From *Hip on Health: Health Information for Caregivers and Families* by Charlotte M. Hendricks. Published by Redleaf Press. www.redleafpress.org.

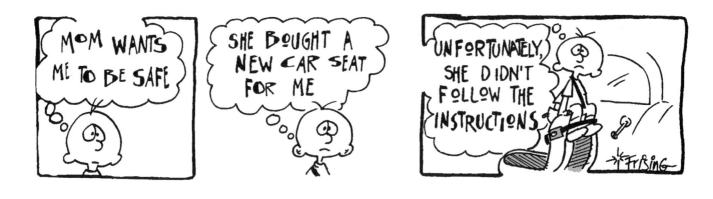

Buckle Up

Motor vehicle accidents are a leading cause of injury and death for young children. A crash at just five miles per hour can throw an unbuckled child into the dashboard or windshield.

Infants and children should use safety seats (car seats) that meet federal motor vehicle safety standards. Infants and children under age two should be securely buckled into safety seats that face the rear of the car. Older toddlers and small children can be buckled into forward-facing safety seats. Older, bigger children should use booster seats along with lap belts and shoulder harnesses.

Find out if the safety seat is designed for the size and age of the child. Follow the instructions carefully when using a safety seat. It should be buckled in tightly so that it does not move more than an inch in any direction on the car seat.

The back seat of the vehicle is the safest place for children. If a vehicle has air bags, never place a safety seat on the front passenger side! Children should not ride in the front seat with an air bag until they are at least twelve years old and tall enough to wear a regular lap-and-shoulder belt properly. Always move the seat back as far as possible.

Children are more likely to buckle up if they see you do so. Teach them to always buckle up and ride the safe way.

Exclusion from Child Care

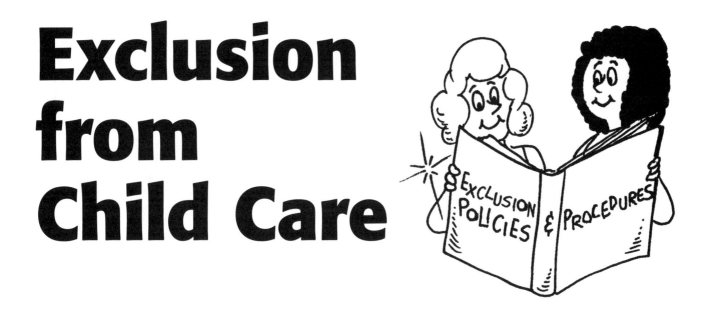

Temporary exclusion from child care because of illness is to prevent the spread of disease.

Children may have minor symptoms of illness, such as runny noses. If they feel well enough to participate in daily activities, they may be allowed to attend child care.

Children's illnesses may require extra care. When caregivers cannot provide this extra care, along with quality care for other enrolled children, ill children should be excluded until their condition improves.

Highly contagious diseases, such as chicken pox, measles, mumps, and diphtheria, require exclusion until the child can no longer infect others.

From *Hip on Health: Health Information for Caregivers and Families* by Charlotte M. Hendricks. Published by Redleaf Press. www.redleafpress.org.

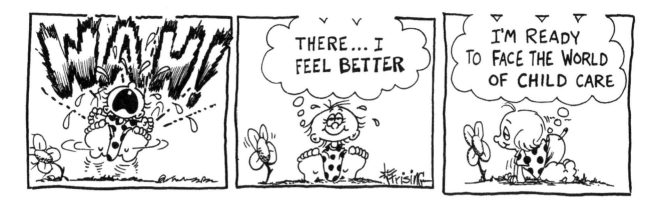

Exclusion from Child Care

When children play with other children in child care, in school, and in the neighborhood, they share germs. That means they occasionally get sick. This brings up the question—may a child with symptoms of illness attend child care or school?

Temporary exclusion from child care because of illness is to prevent the spread of disease and to ensure that all children receive quality care and attention.

Children may have minor symptoms of illness, such as low fever, coughing, or runny nose. If they feel well enough to participate in daily activities, they may be allowed to attend child care. Children who do not feel well should stay home.

Children's conditions or illnesses may require extra care and attention by their caregivers. Caregivers may not have the time and ability to provide this extra care, while also providing high quality care to other children. If so, then ill children should be excluded until their condition improves.

Some illnesses and conditions, such as fever with listlessness, aching, vomiting or diarrhea, and rashes, do require exclusion from child care.

Some illnesses can be treated with medication. For example, a child with strep throat can return to child care twenty-four hours after antibiotic treatment begins. Children with head lice or pinworms can return to child care once appropriate treatment is given.

Some communicable illnesses require exclusion. Whooping cough, chicken pox, measles, mumps, and diphtheria are highly contagious. A doctor or other health care provider should determine when children can return to child care.

Child care programs differ in their exclusion policies for illness. Parents and caregivers should discuss the policy when children are enrolled.

Remember, children occasionally get sick. Try to have backup plans for child care when children become ill.

From *Hip on Health: Health Information for Caregivers and Families* by Charlotte M. Hendricks. Published by Redleaf Press. www.redleafpress.org.

Field Trips

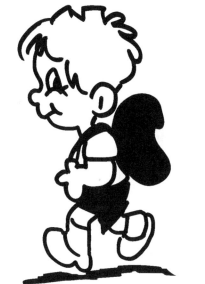

Ask about safety precautions before children are allowed to go on field trips.

- **Where will the children go? What will they do there?**

- **What time will they leave and return?**

- **What transportation will be used?**

- **Will there be enough adults to watch the children?**

- **What if a child gets sick or injured?**

Talk with children before the outing. Discuss where they will go and review safety rules.

From Hip on Health: Health Information for Caregivers and Families by Charlotte M. Hendricks. Published by Redleaf Press. www.redleafpress.org.

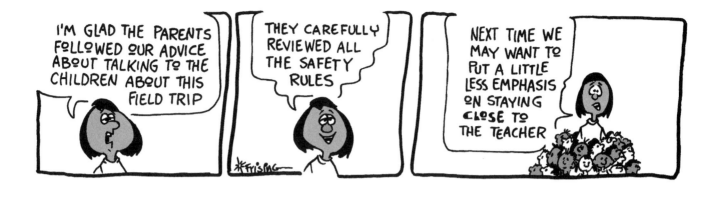

Field Trips

Field trips allow children to experience new sights, places, and activities. Do you worry if they go on a field trip or an outing without you? Ask their teacher about safety precautions before you allow children to go on a field trip. Here are some examples:

✓ Where will the children go? Why are they going? What will they do there?

✓ What time will they leave and return?

✓ What transportation will be used? Will each child have a safety seat?

✓ Have safety seats been properly installed and checked?

✓ Who will be driving? What type of vehicle?

✓ Who will supervise the children? Will there be enough adults to watch them?

✓ What happens when children become sick or injured? Will a first aid kit and medical consent forms be made available? How will parents or guardians be contacted?

Talk with children before the outing. Discuss where they will go and the fun they will have. Review safety rules such as the following:

✓ Stay with the teacher.

✓ Buckle up in the vehicle.

✓ Stay where you are if you get lost.

These discussions can help everyone relax and enjoy the outing.

From *Hip on Health: Health Information for Caregivers and Families* by Charlotte M. Hendricks. Published by Redleaf Press. www.redleafpress.org.

Selecting Child Care

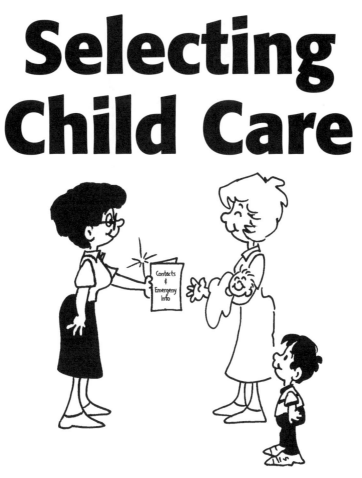

Make sure caregivers have the information necessary to take good care of children. Find out what training and experience they possess. Do they know what to do if children are sick, injured, or choking?

Discuss rules and expectations, such as what to feed children, discipline methods, and nap time.

Leave phone numbers and locations where you and other responsible adults can be reached. Provide phone numbers for the doctor and dentist.

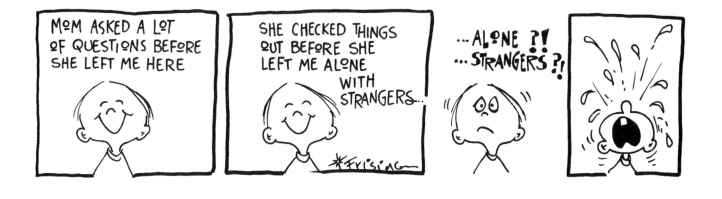

Selecting Child Care

One sign of a good child care program is caregivers who welcome questions and invite you to visit at any time. Here are questions you may want to ask:

✓ How many caregivers are there for the children? Do they hire a substitute when a regular caregiver is absent?

✓ What foods are served for breakfast, lunch, and snack? When are meals and snacks offered?

✓ Do all the children take naps? How long do they sleep? Do all children have their own cribs or cots? What happens when a child does not want to sleep?

✓ How do caregivers manage children's behavior? Spanking should *never* be used in a child care program.

✓ Do the children go on field trips? What transportation is provided? Do they use safety seats?

✓ How safe is the building? Are electric outlets covered? Are cleaning supplies and medicines stored in locked cabinets?

✓ How safe is the play area? Is the play area secured with a fence and latched gate? Is the play equipment safe and age appropriate?

✓ Do caregivers watch the children carefully when playing? Are there soft surfaces under all play equipment?

✓ Are children allowed to attend the program when they are sick? What happens if a child becomes sick or injured while in child care?

Answers to these and other questions can help you assess the quality of care your child will receive. Visit the program unannounced to see how the children are cared for.

From *Hip on Health: Health Information for Caregivers and Families* by Charlotte M. Hendricks. Published by Redleaf Press. www.redleafpress.org.

Sharing Information

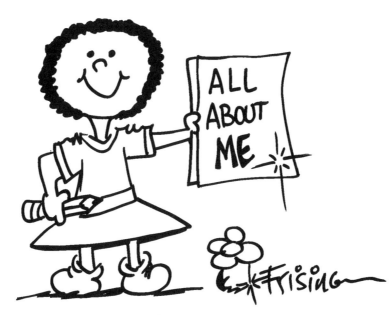

Many children are in child care for 8 or more hours each day. Caregivers can tell parents what their children like to eat, help with toilet training, and provide love and nurturing.

Caregivers also notice changes in children's actions or appearance that might indicate illness, pain, stress, or need for more sleep.

Parents and caregivers should talk to each other daily. Sharing information helps everyone provide the very best care for children!

From *Hip on Health: Health Information for Caregivers and Families* by Charlotte M. Hendricks. Published by Redleaf Press. www.redleafpress.org.

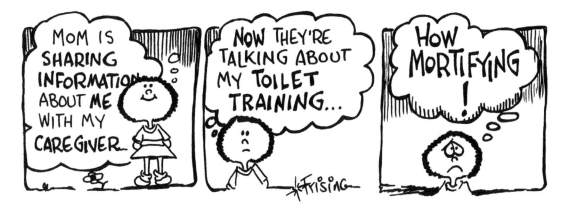

Sharing Information

Many children are in child care for eight or more hours each day. Caregivers can tell parents what their children like to eat, help with toilet training, and provide love and nurturing. Caregivers also notice changes that might indicate illness, pain, stress, or need for more sleep. Caregivers and parents should talk to each other each day.

Parents should share important information about their children. Here are some examples:

✓ diagnosed special needs

✓ chronic medical conditions, such as asthma or diabetes, and written information on how the condition is managed

✓ immunization records

✓ information about allergies and a list of foods, ingredients, chemicals, insect stings, or other substances that may affect the child

✓ changes in children's home life, such as divorce or marriage, new baby in the house, or changes in children's routines

By sharing information, parents and caregivers can provide love, attention, and the very best care for children.

From Hip on Health: Health Information for Caregivers and Families by Charlotte M. Hendricks. Published by Redleaf Press. www.redleafpress.org.

Supplies for Child Care

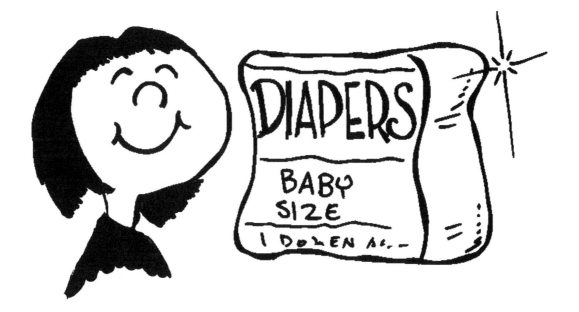

Nutritious food, clean clothing, and children's favorite blankets or toys are all important in daily child care.

Parents and caregivers should discuss which items parents should provide and which ones caregivers will stock.

If parents provide supplies, children should each have a cubby or locker for their personal items. Parents should check children's cubbies and lockers regularly and replenish supplies as needed.

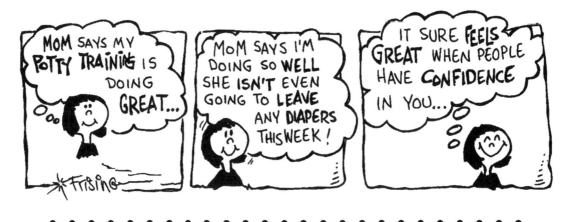

Supplies for Child Care

Parents want their children's needs met each day. Nutritious food, clean clothing, and favorite blankets or toys are all important.

Whether a child is enrolled in a child care center, is in family child care, or stays with a nanny, parents and caregivers should know what each will provide. For example, some child care programs provide food for toddlers and preschoolers but require parents to provide formula and baby food for infants. A caregiver may provide wipes but expect parents to provide diapers.

If parents provide supplies, then each child should have a cubby or locker for personal supplies. Parents should check their children's cubby or locker regularly and replenish supplies as needed.

Here are examples of items that parents or caregivers may provide:

✓ infant formula or breast milk, clean bottles and nipples

✓ prepared baby foods

✓ diapers and wipes

✓ extra clothing, including underwear, shorts, sweats, T-shirts, jackets, and socks

✓ nap time mat and/or blanket

✓ sunscreen (SPF 30)

From *Hip on Health: Health Information for Caregivers and Families* by Charlotte M. Hendricks. Published by Redleaf Press. www.redleafpress.org.

Cold Sores

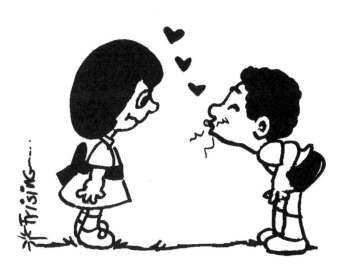

Cold sores are tiny blisters that can form in patches on and around the lips. Children can get cold sores by eating or drinking from the same utensils or by getting kissed by someone who is infected with the Herpes simplex virus (HSV-1).

Cold sores are contagious. Try to prevent spreading the virus by using these precautions:

- Keep drinking glasses, eating utensils, washcloths, and towels of people with cold sores separate.

- Teach children to "blow kisses" to avoid direct contact.

- Wash hands after touching cold sores.

- Teach children to avoid touching cold sores and then touching other areas of their faces. If HSV-1 infects the eyes, it can be serious.

From *Hip on Health: Health Information for Caregivers and Families* by Charlotte M. Hendricks. Published by Redleaf Press. www.redleafpress.org.

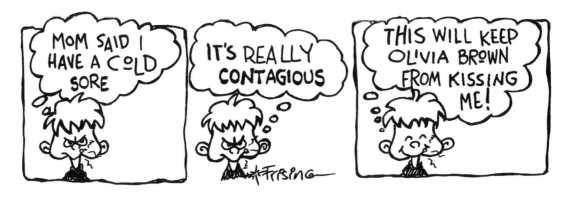

Cold Sores

Cold sores, also called fever blisters, can occur in patches on and around the lips. After the blisters break, a crust forms over the sore. Most cold sores are caused by Herpes simplex virus type 1 (HSV-1). Children can get infected by eating or drinking from the same utensils or by getting kissed by a person with the infection. Cold sores are most contagious when they are oozing fluid.

After children are infected, the virus can lie dormant without causing any symptoms. But it can reactivate later, typically after stress to their bodies. Cold sores might appear when a child has another infection or fever, after exposure to sunlight or cold weather, during menstrual periods, or before a big test at school.

A pharmacist or other health care provider may recommend medicine to shorten the outbreak and make cold sores less painful. Cold sores usually heal in about a week. Call a doctor when children have the following conditions:

✓ weakened immune systems, which could allow the HSV infection to infect other parts of their bodies

✓ sores that do not heal within seven to ten days

✓ sores near their eyes or on their faces

✓ cold sores frequently

HSV-1 is very contagious. Take the following actions to prevent spreading the virus to others:

✓ Keep drinking glasses, eating utensils, washcloths, and towels of people who are infected separate from those used by others. Wash items thoroughly after use.

✓ Teach children to "blow a kiss" to avoid direct contact.

✓ Infected persons and those caring for infected children should wash their hands frequently and immediately after touching cold sores.

✓ Teach children to avoid touching cold sores and then touching other areas of their faces. If HSV-1 infects the eyes, it can be very serious.

From *Hip on Health: Health Information for Caregivers and Families* by Charlotte M. Hendricks. Published by Redleaf Press. www.redleafpress.org.

Fluoride

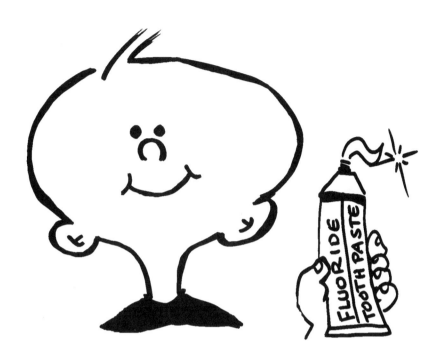

Fluoride helps keep teeth strong and hard. Just a small amount of fluoride helps prevent tooth decay and cavities.

Fluoride is added to many communities' water supplies. Most toothpastes also contain fluoride.

Children (and adults) should brush their teeth daily with fluoride toothpaste. A tiny smear on the toothbrush is enough.

Children should visit a dentist every 6 months. Ask about fluoride treatments.

From *Hip on Health: Health Information for Caregivers and Families* by Charlotte M. Hendricks. Published by Redleaf Press. www.redleafpress.org.

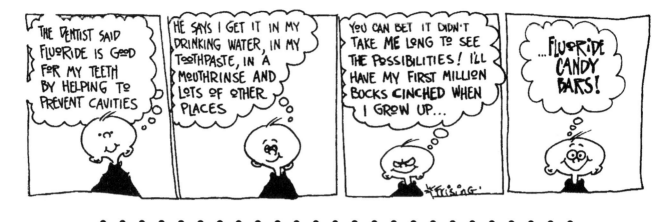

Fluoride

Fluoride is a natural element found in water, soil, and many foods and beverages. Fluoride helps keep teeth strong and hard. Just a small amount helps prevent tooth decay and cavities.

Here are some ways children can get fluoride:

✓ Fluoride is often added to communities' water supplies. This gives dental protection with every drink of water. Most bottled waters do *not* contain fluoride.

✓ Most toothpastes contain fluoride. Help children brush teeth daily using fluoride toothpaste. A tiny smear of toothpaste is enough to use for brushing.

✓ Some mouth rinses contain fluoride. Older children can use these products to swish and spit. Children under age six should not use mouth rinse because they may swallow it instead of spitting it out.

✓ Fluoride drops or tablets may be prescribed by a doctor or dentist.

Dentists may offer fluoride treatments. Fluoride gel may be put into a plastic mouthpiece that children hold in their mouths for a few minutes. Some dentists have children brush their teeth with a fluoride toothpaste. Others may paint children's teeth with clear fluoride.

Children should visit a dentist as soon as the first tooth appears or by their first birthday. Checkups should occur every six months.

From *Hip on Health: Health Information for Caregivers and Families* by Charlotte M. Hendricks. Published by Redleaf Press. www.redleafpress.org.

Preventing Dental Injury

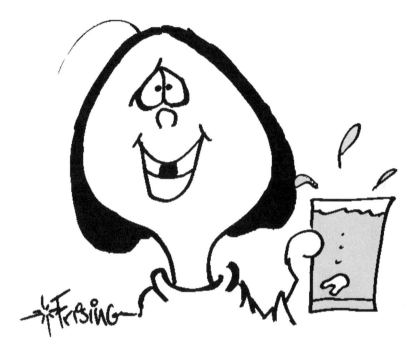

All teeth are important! You can help protect children's teeth from injury.

Toddlers and young children often fall or bump into furniture as they learn to walk and explore their environment. They may hit their mouths and loosen their front teeth.

Keep pathways clear for walking. Use safety gates at stairways. Pad the edges of low furniture, such as coffee tables.

From *Hip on Health: Health Information for Caregivers and Families* by Charlotte M. Hendricks. Published by Redleaf Press. www.redleafpress.org.

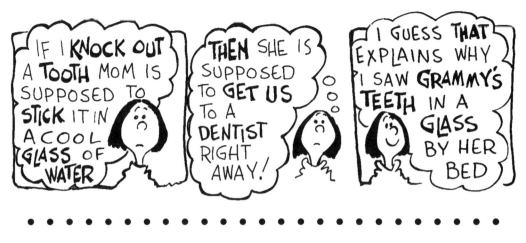

Preventing Dental Injury

All teeth are important—even primary (baby) teeth. You can help protect children's teeth from injury.

Toddlers and young children often fall or bump into furniture as they learn to walk and explore. They may hit their mouths and loosen their front teeth.

Keep pathways clear for walking. Use safety gates at stairways. Pad the edges of low furniture, such as coffee tables.

Older children may injure their teeth when skateboarding, in-line skating, or bicycling. Insist that children wear helmets to prevent dental and head injuries. Helmets should fit children's heads snugly and cover their foreheads. If children fall, their helmets—not their foreheads—will hit the ground first and hold their faces (and teeth) away from the ground.

If teeth become loosened or knocked out, take the child to a dentist immediately—within an hour, if possible. The dentist may be able to save the teeth.

If a tooth becomes broken or knocked out, collect all of its pieces. If it's dirty, rinse it gently in clean running water, but do not scrub it. Place the tooth in a wet cloth or in a container of water or milk. For an older child, if there is no danger that he or she will swallow the tooth, you may gently put it back in its socket and hold it in place.

From *Hip on Health: Health Information for Caregivers and Families* by Charlotte M. Hendricks. Published by Redleaf Press. www.redleafpress.org.

Teething

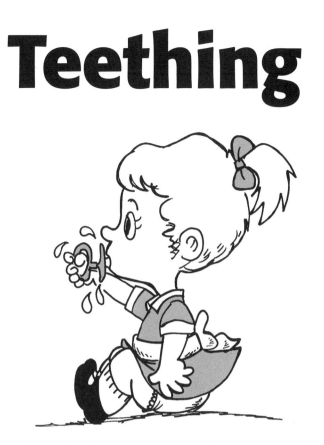

Teething usually begins between 6 and 12 months and continues until the child is about 3 years old. Here are some ways to soothe teething children:

- Distract them with extra attention, playtime, music, or special toys.

- Wipe their faces and chins often to remove drool.

- Give them something to chew on, such as a cold wet cloth or rubber teething ring.

- Rub infants' gums with your clean finger.

From *Hip on Health: Health Information for Caregivers and Families* by Charlotte M. Hendricks. Published by Redleaf Press. www.redleafpress.org.

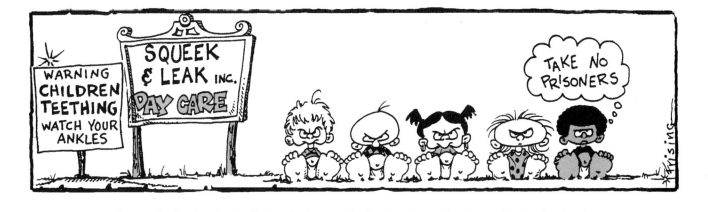

Teething

Teething usually begins between six and twelve months and continues until children are about three years old.

Teething children may drool, chew on their fingers or toys, or have trouble sleeping or eating because of pain. They may have swollen and red gums or small red or white spots on their gums. They may be irritable and cranky while teething.

Here are some ways to soothe teething infants:

✓ Distract them with extra attention, playtime, music, or toys.

✓ Wipe their faces and chins often to remove drool.

✓ Give them cold wet cloths or rubber teething rings to chew.

✓ Rub infants' gums with your clean finger.

✓ Give cold foods (applesauce, yogurt, or baby food) or warm soft foods (mashed vegetables or baby cereals) that may feel good on sore gums.

Do not place teething rings in the freezer; frozen rings can damage teeth. Avoid liquid-filled teething rings, which can break. Avoid teething crackers; these may cause choking.

Teething gels generally are not recommended. Too much gel can numb infants' mouths and cause difficulty swallowing or breathing. *Never* give aspirin, paregoric, or alcoholic beverages.

If children's doctors recommend pain relievers such as acetaminophen or ibuprofen, ask a pharmacist to help you choose the correct type and dosage for children's weight and age. Do not give aspirin to children.

From *Hip on Health: Health Information for Caregivers and Families* by Charlotte M. Hendricks. Published by Redleaf Press. www.redleafpress.org.

Tooth Brushing

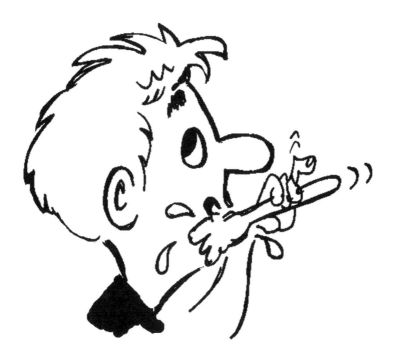

Help children brush their teeth at least twice each day. Brushing removes food particles and helps prevent tooth decay and gum disease. Here are some tips for effective tooth brushing:

- Use soft, child-size toothbrushes.

- Use just a tiny smear of fluoride toothpaste.

- Gently wiggle and sweep the bristles over the teeth and gums.

- Brush the tongue.

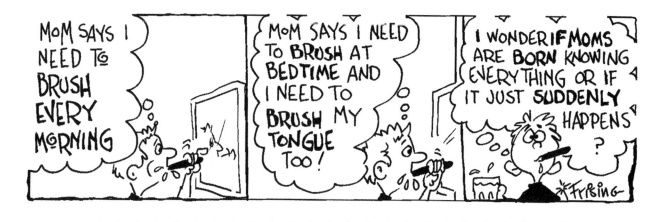

Tooth Brushing

Children should brush their teeth at least twice a day. The most important time to brush is at bedtime. If food particles and bacteria stay on the teeth, they can cause tooth decay, gum problems, and bad breath.

Young children need your help with tooth brushing. Here are some tips:

✓ Use soft, child-size toothbrushes. Replace them every three months or when they look worn.

✓ For children over two years, choose toothpaste with fluoride. Use just a tiny smear of toothpaste.

✓ Place the brush at an angle against the teeth and gently wiggle and sweep the bristles over the teeth and gums.

✓ Brush the tongue.

✓ Rinse toothbrushes thoroughly and air-dry them.

Begin helping children learn to floss when they have two teeth that touch each other.

✓ Guide the floss between the teeth, using a gentle rubbing motion.

✓ When the floss reaches the gum line, curve it into a *C* shape against one tooth.

✓ Gently rub the side of the tooth, moving the floss away from the gum with up and down motions.

Children should first visit the dentist when they are about one year old or before then if you notice any problems with their mouths or teeth.

From *Hip on Health: Health Information for Caregivers and Families* by Charlotte M. Hendricks. Published by Redleaf Press. www.redleafpress.org.

Tooth Care for Infants

Clean infants' gums and teeth after every feeding, especially before bedtime.

Wash your hands thoroughly.

Use your finger to gently wipe a soft damp cloth or gauze over infants' gums after feeding.

Gently massage the gums.

Once children's teeth are showing, brush them with very soft, tiny infants' toothbrushes and plain water. Do not use toothpaste.

From *Hip on Health: Health Information for Caregivers and Families* by Charlotte M. Hendricks. Published by Redleaf Press. www.redleafpress.org.

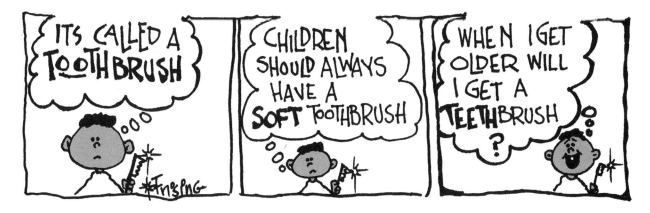

Tooth Care for Infants

Good oral health begins with prevention—before the first tooth appears. Clean infants' gums and teeth after every feeding, especially before bedtime.

Clean infants' gums and teeth in this way:

✓ Wash your hands thoroughly.

✓ Use your finger to gently wipe a soft damp cloth or gauze over infants' gums after feeding. Gently massage the gums.

✓ Once infant's teeth are showing, brush them with very soft, tiny infants' toothbrushes and plain water. *Do not* use toothpaste.

✓ Clean and massage the gums where there are no teeth.

When formula, breast milk, or other sweet liquids are available to children in bottles or cups throughout the day or night, tooth decay can occur. Usually, the front teeth are damaged.

✓ Do not allow infants to suck on bottles or cups between meals.

✓ Never give pacifiers sweetened with honey, corn syrup, or other sweet liquids.

✓ Do not allow infants to take bottles to bed.

✓ Wean infants from bottles as soon as they can hold cups.

From *Hip on Health: Health Information for Caregivers and Families* by Charlotte M. Hendricks. Published by Redleaf Press. www.redleafpress.org.

Sealants

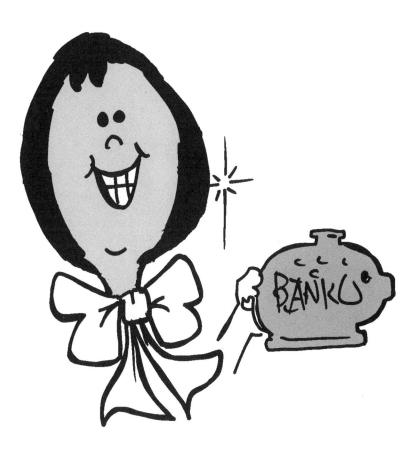

The surfaces of the back teeth (molars) have deep grooves and ridges. Dentists may apply thin plastic coverings to the top chewing surfaces of healthy back teeth. These dental sealants cover and seal the grooves to prevent cavities.

Sealants are usually applied when children are 6 to 12 years old. Sealants can stay on and protect teeth for many years.

From *Hip on Health: Health Information for Caregivers and Families* by Charlotte M. Hendricks. Published by Redleaf Press. www.redleafpress.org.

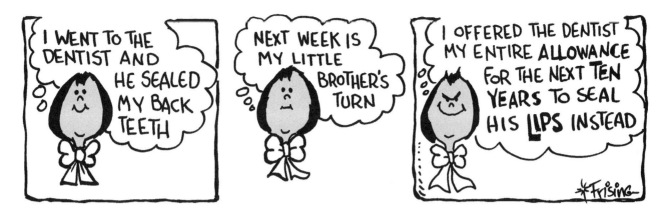

Sealants

Dentists can help prevent cavities by putting dental sealants on children's teeth.

Dental sealants are thin plastic covers placed on the chewing surfaces of healthy teeth. The surfaces of the back teeth (molars) have deep grooves and ridges. Food and plaque can become stuck in these grooves and cause tooth decay. The sealant covers and seals these grooves to keep food out, preventing cavities.

Sealants should be applied to children's permanent molars as soon as they come in. Sealants are usually applied when children are six to twelve years old. It takes only a few minutes to apply them. This is how they work:

✓ Dentists clean the surface of each tooth and may put gauze around the tooth to keep it dry.

✓ They paint a liquid on the tooth to help the sealant stick.

✓ Next, they paint the tooth with the sealant material. The liquid sealant flows into the grooves of the tooth and then hardens to form a white or clear plastic covering.

✓ Dentists may use a special light to harden the sealant.

Children do not feel or see the sealants on the teeth. Sealants should stay on and protect teeth for many years. Dentists can check to be sure existing sealants are still sealed properly.

Cuts and Wounds

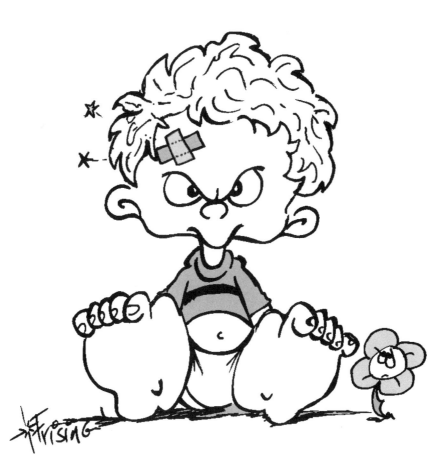

Most small cuts and scrapes heal by themselves.

Clean wounds with mild soap and water. Parents can apply an antibiotic ointment and a bandage.

Watch for signs of infection. Call the child's doctor if the wound becomes red, swollen, tender, warm, or begins to drain.

From *Hip on Health: Health Information for Caregivers and Families* by Charlotte M. Hendricks. Published by Redleaf Press. www.redleafpress.org.

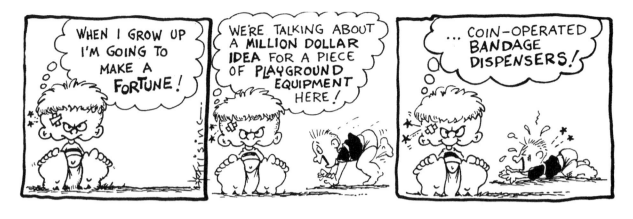

Cuts and Wounds

Children get plenty of cuts, scratches, and scrapes. With a little first aid, you can usually kiss away the hurt. Follow these steps:

✓ Apply firm direct pressure on wounds to stop bleeding.

✓ Clean wounds thoroughly with mild soap and water.

✓ Cover wounds. Children love colorful bandages!

✓ When bandages get wet, remove them and apply new ones. After wounds form scabs, bandages are no longer necessary.

Antibiotic ointment or cream may promote healing and prevent infection. Watch for signs of infection. Call the child's doctor if the wound becomes red, swollen, tender, warm, or begins to drain.

Large or deep wounds can be serious. If blood is spurting out or wounds are large and bleeding severely, call 911! Call the child's doctor if the following occurs:

✓ A wound does not stop bleeding after five minutes of direct pressure. If blood is spurting out, call 911!

✓ The cut seems deep, is more than ½ inch long, or will not stay closed by itself. Deep cuts can damage underlying nerves and tendons.

✓ The wound is on the child's face or neck or affects the eyes, ears, or lips.

✓ Something is stuck in the wound or it cannot be cleaned of dirt and debris thoroughly.

✓ The wound is from a bite (animal or human).

From *Hip on Health: Health Information for Caregivers and Families* by Charlotte M. Hendricks. Published by Redleaf Press. www.redleafpress.org.

Disaster Preparation

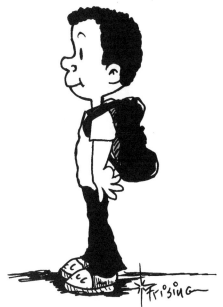

Natural events, such as tornado, hurricane, earthquake, fire, blizzard, and flood, can lead to emergency situations. Early childhood programs must be prepared. The staff should be able to answer questions like these:

- Does the program have written policy and procedures?

- Do staff and children regularly practice drills?

- Does the program have a tornado-safe area?

- How will children be transported if evacuation is required?

Teachers should have current contact information for parents.

From *Hip on Health: Health Information for Caregivers and Families* by Charlotte M. Hendricks. Published by Redleaf Press. www.redleafpress.org.

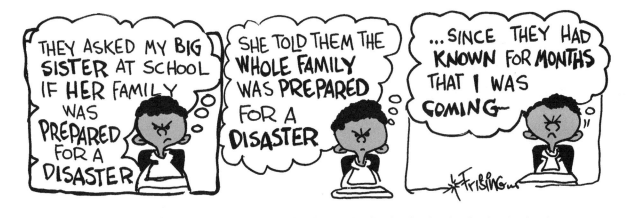

Disaster Preparation

The threat of emergency or disaster has always been with us. Tornado, hurricane, fire, blizzard, earthquake, or flood can lead to emergency situations.

Make sure that the staff of children's early childhood programs are prepared for emergencies. They should be able to answer questions like these:

✓ Are there written policies and procedures for emergencies?

✓ Are there two exits from every room?

✓ How will infants and toddlers be evacuated?

✓ Is there a tornado-safe area?

✓ Is there an off-site safe shelter in case evacuation is necessary?

✓ How will children be transported in an emergency?

✓ Is there a lockdown procedure in place for potentially violent situations?

✓ Do staff and children regularly practice drills?

✓ Are "ready-to-go" files with contact information available for each child?

✓ Is extra food and water available on-site?

Make sure children's caregivers and teachers have current contact information for parents and other responsible adults, including home, work, and cell numbers.

From *Hip on Health: Health Information for Caregivers and Families* by Charlotte M. Hendricks. Published by Redleaf Press. www.redleafpress.org.

Emergency Help

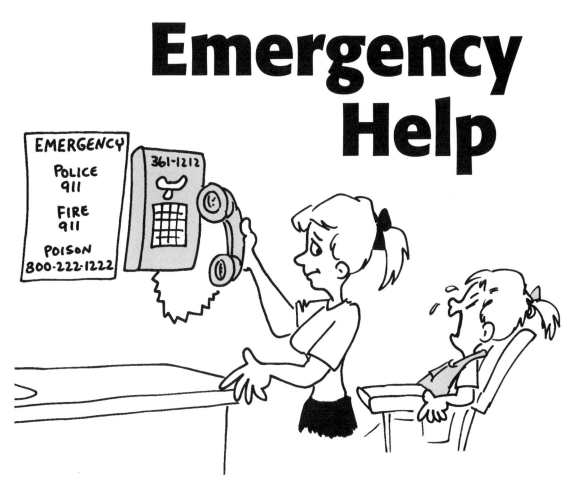

What happens when a child becomes injured or starts choking? Do you know first aid and rescue breathing? Do you know how to get emergency help?

A child can sustain permanent brain damage or die in just a few minutes from bleeding, breathing problems, or poisoning.

Put the emergency number (911) and the Poison Control Center number (1-800-222-1222) on every telephone.

The best treatment for injury is prevention.

From *Hip on Health: Health Information for Caregivers and Families* by Charlotte M. Hendricks. Published by Redleaf Press. www.redleafpress.org.

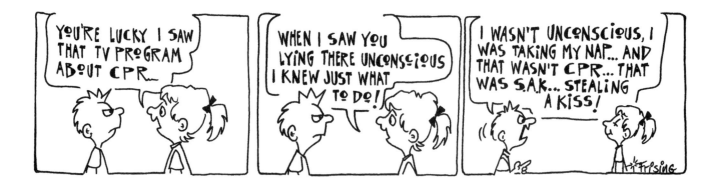

Emergency Help

Sometimes you need emergency help. Three emergency cases are bleeding, breathing, and poisoning.

Bleeding: A child can bleed to death in less than a minute if a large blood vein or artery is cut. If a child is bleeding, apply direct pressure to stop it. If you cannot immediately control the bleeding by direct pressure or if blood spurts out, **call 911!**

Breathing: A child who is not breathing can sustain permanent brain damage in four minutes. If a child cannot cough, speak, or breathe, **call 911!** If the child is having difficulty breathing and lips, skin, or fingernails look "bluish," he or she is not getting enough oxygen. **Call 911!**

Poisoning: Poisons that are eaten or breathed in can be deadly in just a few minutes. If you think a child has swallowed or breathed poison, call the **Poison Control Center at 1-800-222-1222**. You will be told what to do.

Injuries or illnesses can be serious. Children who have suffered head, neck, or back injuries or burns need immediate medical help.

Parents should learn first aid and rescue breathing or CPR. Check with your local American Red Cross, American Heart Association, health department, or hospital to learn about courses offered in your area.

The best treatment for childhood injury is prevention!

From *Hip on Health: Health Information for Caregivers and Families* by Charlotte M. Hendricks. Published by Redleaf Press. www.redleafpress.org.

First Aid Kit

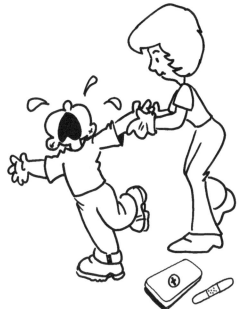

Often, a colorful bandage can stop a child's tears. Here are other items needed for your first aid kit:

- digital thermometer

- several sizes of bandages

- gauze, tape, and scissors

- tweezers

- medicine spoon

- protective gloves

Take your first aid kit when you travel with children.

From *Hip on Health: Health Information for Caregivers and Families* by Charlotte M. Hendricks. Published by Redleaf Press. www.redleafpress.org.

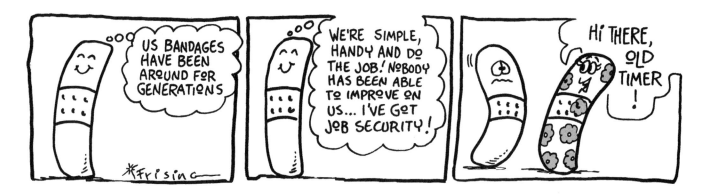

First Aid Kit

Have you noticed how quickly a hug and a kiss make a cut or scrape feel better? Or that a colorful bandage can stop tears?

Here are items you may want to keep in your first aid kit:

- ✓ thermometer—plastic digital type

- ✓ bandages—various sizes and colors

- ✓ gauze, tape, and scissors for larger scrapes or cuts

- ✓ tweezers to remove splinters

- ✓ medicine spoon to accurately measure medicine doses

- ✓ protective gloves to avoid touching blood and body fluids

- ✓ facecloth to clean skin or make a soft ice pack

- ✓ plastic zipper bags to make ice packs or dispose of used bandages

- ✓ premoistened towelettes to clean hands or skin

Take your first aid kit with you when you travel.

If you include medicine in your kit, remember that it should not be left in a vehicle where it can get too hot or cold. Keep all medicines out of children's sight and out of reach!

From *Hip on Health: Health Information for Caregivers and Families* by Charlotte M. Hendricks. Published by Redleaf Press. www.redleafpress.org.

Teach Children Their Names and Addresses

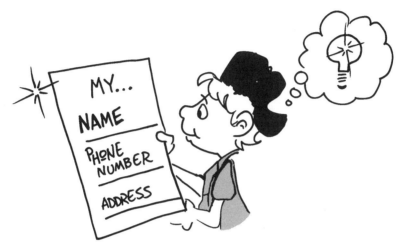

Talk to children about who is allowed to pick them up from school or take them somewhere. Help children learn the names of these people.

Teach children what to do if someone else tries to take them. They should yell and scream, "You are not my mommy (or daddy)."

Explain that if they become lost, cannot find you, or are scared, they can go to a police officer, store clerk, or another parent with children. These people can help find you.

From *Hip on Health: Health Information for Caregivers and Families* by Charlotte M. Hendricks. Published by Redleaf Press. www.redleafpress.org.

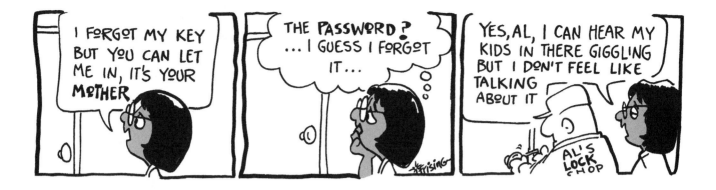

Teach Children Their Names and Addresses

Most young children like to talk. It is important to teach them to say their names, addresses, and phone numbers. Begin by teaching them to say their first and last name. Next, they can learn to say their parents' or guardians' names.

When learning addresses and phone numbers, children may find it easier to "sing" or say them in a fun way. Help them practice saying these in the car, at bedtime, or during meals.

Tell children that if they become lost or need help, they can give their names and addresses to a police officer, firefighter, store clerk, or another parent with children. These are people who can help find you.

When children become lost or cannot find you in a store or other place, they should stay in that store and ask someone to help find you. They should never leave the store or go into the parking lot to find you. Tell them that you will be looking for them!

Talk to children about whom you trust to take care of them, to pick them up from school, or to take them somewhere. Help them learn the names of these people.

Teach children what to do if someone else tries to take them. They should yell and scream, "You are not my mommy (or daddy)."

From *Hip on Health: Health Information for Caregivers and Families* by Charlotte M. Hendricks. Published by Redleaf Press. www.redleafpress.org.

Bed Wetting

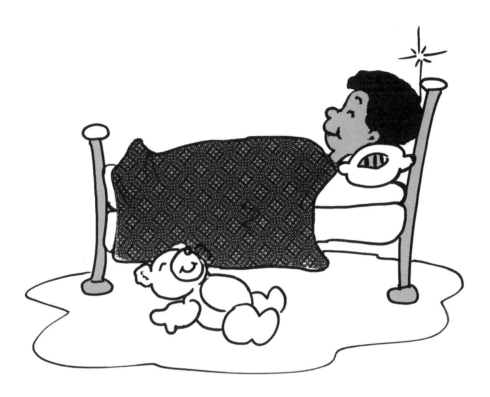

Nighttime bed wetting is very common among young children. Many children who are dry (toilet trained) during the day may still wet the bed.

Be sensitive to children's feelings about bed wetting. Set a no-teasing rule.

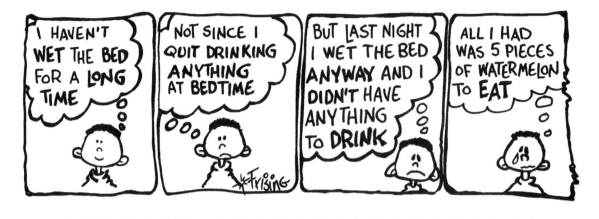

Bed Wetting

Nighttime bed wetting is very common among young children. Many children who are dry (toilet trained) during the day may still wet the bed.

Sometimes children who have been dry at night start bed wetting again. There are many reasons they may wet the bed. Stress in their lives, such as a new baby or moving, can cause bed wetting. Medications, especially those that cause drowsiness, can make children sleep more soundly and wet their beds. Illness also can cause problems. Children who are being physically or sexually abused may start bed wetting.

Do not worry about occasional bed wetting. However, if children often wet the bed after having been dry at night in the past, talk to their doctors.

Children should use the toilet just before bedtime. Do not give large amounts of fluid an hour or so before bedtime.

If possible, let children help change the sheets and covers, but be sensitive to their feelings about bed wetting. They may be embarrassed or scared that friends will find out. Make sure they understand that bed wetting is not their fault and that it will get better. Set a no-teasing rule.

From *Hip on Health: Health Information for Caregivers and Families* by Charlotte M. Hendricks. Published by Redleaf Press. www.redleafpress.org.

Bedtime and Rest

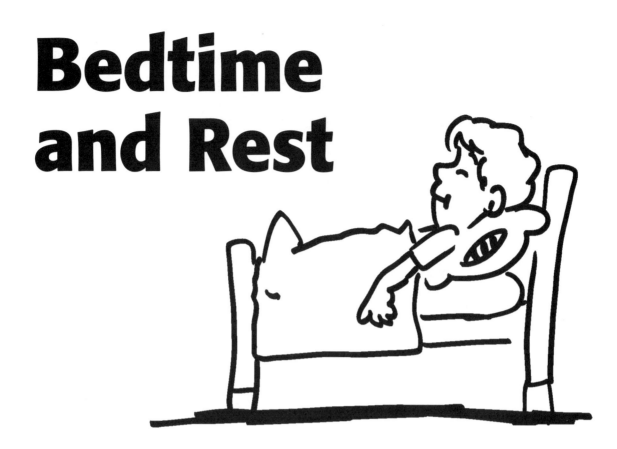

Children need much more sleep than adults.

Infants may sleep as many as 18 hours each day. Toddlers need about 12 hours of sleep each night and 1 or 2 naps during the day.

Preschoolers need 10 to 12 hours of sleep each night and a short nap during the day.

Children fall asleep more quickly when their bedtime routines allow them to relax, such as taking a bath, brushing teeth, reading a story, getting a drink of water, and receiving lots of hugs.

From *Hip on Health: Health Information for Caregivers and Families* by Charlotte M. Hendricks. Published by Redleaf Press. www.redleafpress.org.

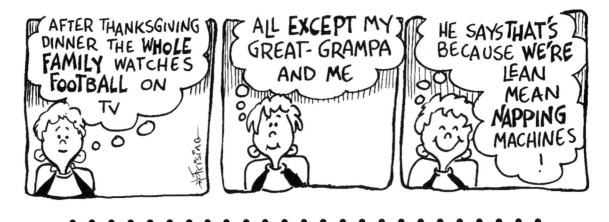

Bedtime and Rest

Do children get enough sleep each night? Do they wake up easily and happily? Do they enjoy playing until it is time to take a nap?

Children need much more sleep than adults. Infants may sleep as many as eighteen hours each day. Toddlers need about twelve hours of sleep each night and one or two naps during the day. Preschoolers need ten to twelve hours of sleep each night and a short nap during the day.

Children need schedules that provide enough sleep. For example, if a four-year-old must awake at 7:00 each morning, then he or she should be in bed by 8:30 each evening. Children should stay on schedule as much as possible during weekends too.

Many children dislike bedtime. Often, the more tired they are, the more they try to stay awake. They fall asleep more quickly when they have routines that allow them to relax before bedtime. Routines may include taking a bath, brushing teeth, listening to a story, getting a drink of water, and receiving lots of hugs.

Some children have difficulty sleeping because of bad dreams. These may be caused by seeing or experiencing violence or a frightening event, watching scary television shows or commercials, and hearing adults talk about frightening events. Even children's stories and fairy tales can be frightening. Bad dreams are very real to children. Hold them close and try to calm them. You may ask what the dream was about. If you know what frightens children, you may be able to prevent bad dreams in the future.

From *Hip on Health: Health Information for Caregivers and Families* by Charlotte M. Hendricks. Published by Redleaf Press. www.redleafpress.org.

Bedtime Routines

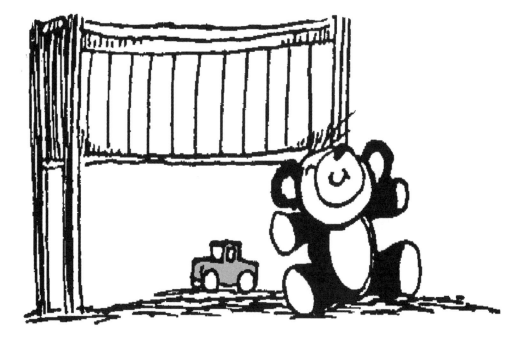

Infants need lots of sleep. Comforting routines help them learn to get themselves to sleep and sleep through the night.

Bedtime routines may include warm baths, singing songs, and reading stories. Hold and snuggle infants, and rock them gently.

Rock infants until they are sleepy but still awake, then put them in their cribs.

From *Hip on Health: Health Information for Caregivers and Families* by Charlotte M. Hendricks. Published by Redleaf Press. www.redleafpress.org.

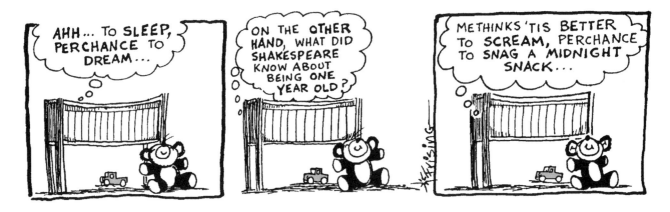

Bedtime Routines

Infants need lots of sleep. Newborns and young infants generally sleep sixteen to twenty hours each day, waking every four or five hours. Infants three to six months old average five hours of sleep during the day and ten hours at night. Most infants wake up once or twice during the night.

Older infants, six to twelve months old, may nap about three hours during the day, and sleep about eleven hours at night.

Comforting bedtime routines help children go to sleep and remain asleep through the night. Give infants warm baths, sing songs, and rock them gently. Hold and snuggle them, and tell a story or read to them.

Infants should sleep in their own cribs. Rock them until they are sleepy but still awake, then put them in their cribs.

Always check on crying infants. If they cry when put in their cribs, check to be sure they are not wet, hungry, sick, hot, or cold. If they appear to be ill, pick them up and comfort them. Call a doctor if necessary.

If they appear to be okay but continue to cry, you should check on them every few minutes. Rub them gently but do not play or turn on bright lights.

If infants continue to cry every night and there does not appear to be anything wrong, let them cry a few minutes before checking on them. For example, let them cry about three minutes before consoling the first night; five minutes the second night, etc. Never allow infants to cry more than ten minutes without trying to comfort them.

From *Hip on Health: Health Information for Caregivers and Families* by Charlotte M. Hendricks. Published by Redleaf Press. www.redleafpress.org.

Dressing for the Weather

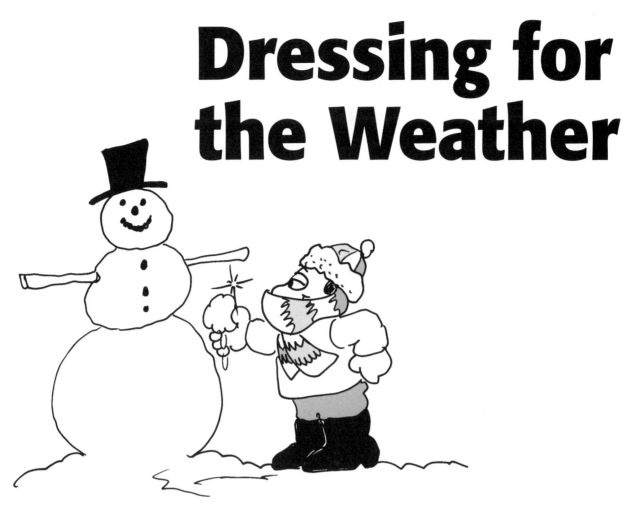

Outdoor play is good for children.

Dress them in layers of clothes that can be removed if they become too warm.

Choose comfortable clothes that children can run, play, and roll in. Remember, play clothes get dirty.

Buy well-fitted shoes good for running and playing. Select closed shoes that tie or strap securely so children won't slip when running.

From *Hip on Health: Health Information for Caregivers and Families* by Charlotte M. Hendricks. Published by Redleaf Press. www.redleafpress.org.

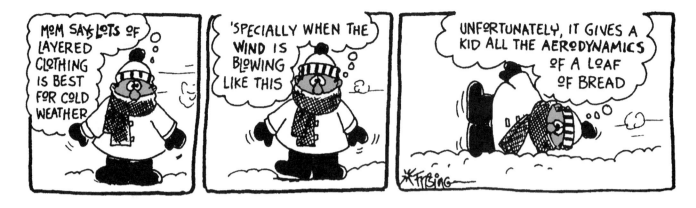

Dressing for the Weather

Children need to run, jump, and be active every day. Except in severe weather, children should play outside each day. Dress them for outdoor play in comfortable clothes. Children like to dig in the dirt and roll in the grass. They need clothes that can get dirty and be washed, such as comfortable pants and pullover shirts.

Buy shoes that fit and protect their feet. Closed shoes with rubber soles, such as sneakers, are best for young children. Sandals, open shoes, and shoes with slick bottoms can cause children to trip and fall. Going barefoot is not safe because children may step on broken glass, nails, or wires, or be bitten by bugs or snakes.

Children can get blisters if shoes rub their skin. Help prevent blisters by getting shoes that fit and tie or strap securely. Wearing socks helps prevent blisters.

Children can play outside even when it is cold. Dress them in layers, including jackets that can be removed if the children become too warm. Despite the cold, children can get hot while running and playing hard.

From *Hip on Health: Health Information for Caregivers and Families* by Charlotte M. Hendricks. Published by Redleaf Press. www.redleafpress.org.

Ears and Hearing

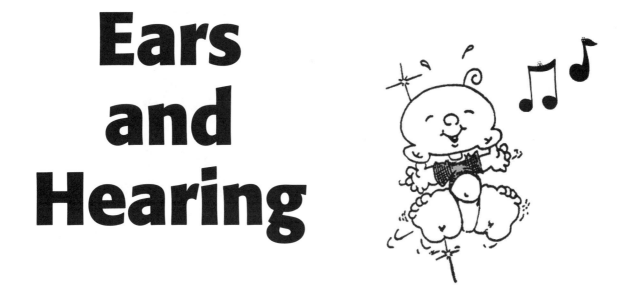

Children with hearing loss may have difficulty communicating, learning, and developing physical skills that require balance. All children should have their hearing checked regularly.

Help children learn to protect their ears and hearing. These precautions will help:

- Keep the volume down on TVs, vehicle stereos, headphones, earbuds, and other devices.

- Make children wear ear protection when around loud machinery, gunfire, or other loud noises.

- Avoid putting anything in children's ears, including cotton swabs.

From *Hip on Health: Health Information for Caregivers and Families* by Charlotte M. Hendricks. Published by Redleaf Press. www.redleafpress.org.

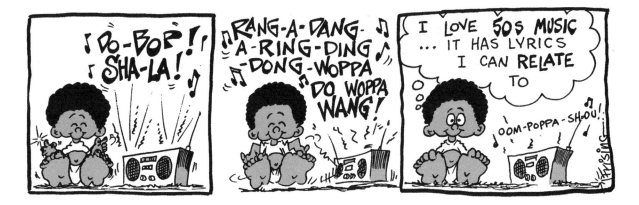

Ears and Hearing

Infants who are born prematurely or have low birth weight may be at risk for hearing problems. Frequent and persistent ear infections and illnesses like mumps can cause hearing loss. Injuries to the ears or head can also cause hearing problems. Hearing problems can also be caused by genetic disorders.

Water in the ears or buildups of ear wax can cause temporary hearing losses. However, do *not* try to clean out children's ears with cotton swabs or other objects. Do *not* use ear drops unless advised by a health care professional.

Children with hearing loss may have difficulty communicating, learning, and developing physical skills that require balance. Infants should have their hearing screened within the first month of life. Older children should have their hearing tested before they enter school, or any time there is a concern about their hearing. Contact their doctor if you suspect hearing loss.

Signs of hearing loss may include the following:

✓ not turning eyes or head toward a sound

✓ poor or limited speech

✓ not following directions or responding to questions or conversations

✓ turning up the volume too high on TV or music devices

Help children learn to protect their ears and hearing. These precautions will help:

✓ Keep the volume down on TVs, vehicle stereos, headphones, earbuds, and other devices.

✓ Make them wear ear protection when around loud machinery, gunfire, or other loud noises.

✓ Avoid putting anything in their ears, including cotton swabs.

From *Hip on Health: Health Information for Caregivers and Families* by Charlotte M. Hendricks. Published by Redleaf Press. www.redleafpress.org.

Eyes and Vision

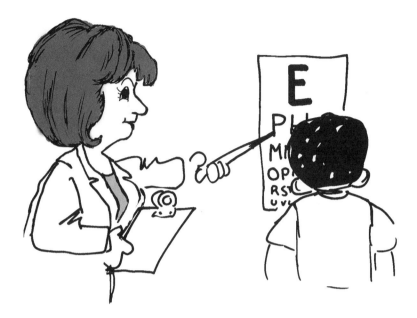

Children should have their eyes and vision checked regularly. Their first full vision checkup may be when they are three years old.

Contact their doctor if you notice that children have any of the following conditions:

- have crossed eyes

- do not seem to see objects clearly

- have crusty, itchy, or red eyes, or their eyes hurt

- have injured their eye(s)

From *Hip on Health: Health Information for Caregivers and Families* by Charlotte M. Hendricks. Published by Redleaf Press. www.redleafpress.org.

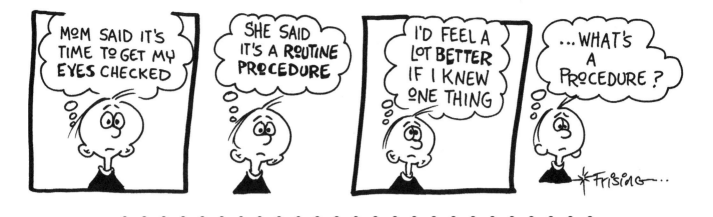

Eyes and Vision

How well do children see? They should have their eyes and vision checked regularly. Infants and very young children have their vision screened during well-child visits. Their first full vision checkups may occur when they are three years old or earlier if they seem to have problems seeing. Children who sit very close to the television set or hold books or objects close to their faces may need glasses.

Red or bloodshot eyes can be caused by infections, allergies, lack of sleep, or dirt in the eye. Call children's doctors if the redness does not clear within a few hours.

Eye problems can be serious. You should call a child's doctor if you notice the following in a child:

✓ does not seem to see objects clearly or has cloudy eyes

✓ has crossed eyes or a wandering eye

✓ has eyes that are crusty, itchy, red, or swollen

✓ complains that his or her eye hurts

Call a doctor immediately when children injure their eyes. Broken glass, sticks, rocks, BB pellets, and other objects can cause serious damage.

The sun's UV rays can also harm young eyes. Encourage children to wear sunglasses labeled "100% UV Protection." Teach them to look away from the sun and other bright lights.

From *Hip on Health: Health Information for Caregivers and Families* by Charlotte M. Hendricks. Published by Redleaf Press. www.redleafpress.org.

Fitness for Children

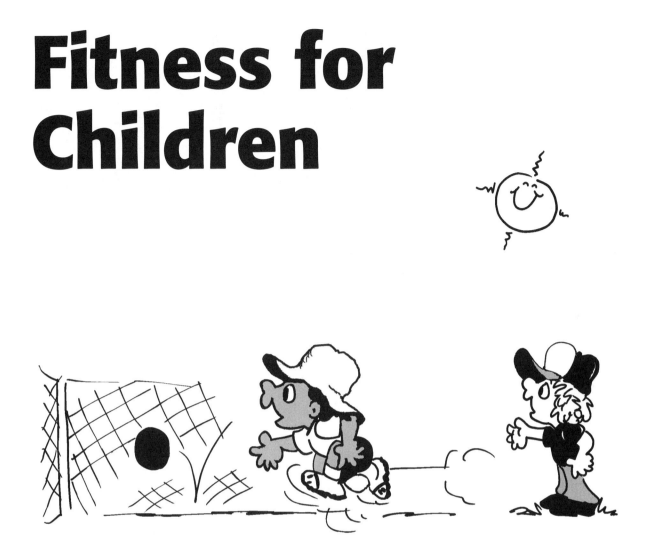

Children need at least one hour of active play each day. Physical activity helps them grow strong and healthy.

Most children like to run, jump, and play.

Be sure they have a safe place to play. Then encourage lots of physical activity.

From *Hip on Health: Health Information for Caregivers and Families* by Charlotte M. Hendricks. Published by Redleaf Press. www.redleafpress.org.

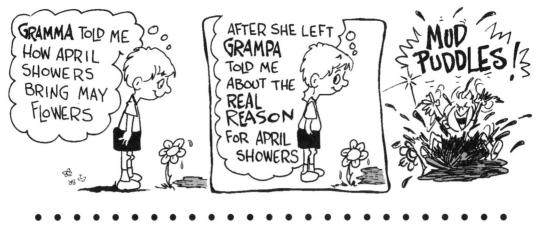

Fitness for Children

Children need at least one hour of active play each day. Physical activity such as running, jumping, crawling, and climbing helps develop strong muscles and bones. Regular physical activity helps young bodies stay healthy and fight germs. Physical activity releases children's energy and relieves stress while they have fun. Overall, children feel better when they are active and moving!

Children naturally like to play, and adults should encourage them. Limit the amount of time they watch TV or play computer games.

Choose a safe place for them to play. Parks and playgrounds may have enclosed areas for play. Always watch children when they are playing outdoors. It is even better if you play with them! Here are some activities young children enjoy:

✓ Softball, soccer, kickball, and catch are fun and help develop motor skills. A plastic or soft bat and big, soft balls are best for young children. Do not keep score. Just have fun!

✓ Sprinklers and water hoses provide cool games for hot summer days.

✓ Running and tag games develop leg muscles.

✓ Rolling down grassy hills or across the lawn can be fun.

✓ Jumping rope helps develop coordination.

From *Hip on Health: Health Information for Caregivers and Families* by Charlotte M. Hendricks. Published by Redleaf Press. www.redleafpress.org.

Growth

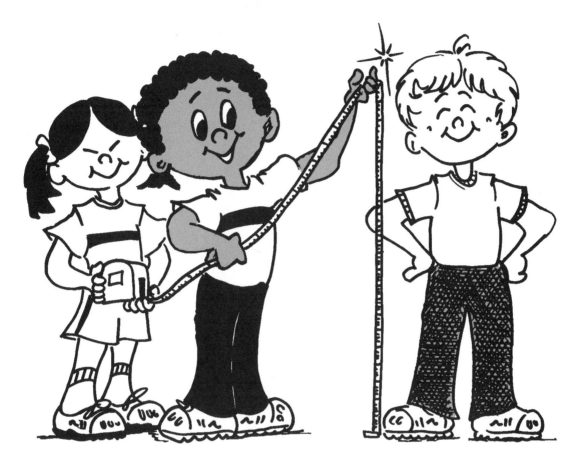

Children grow at different rates. Some children are tall and some children are short. Some children are thin and some are stout. These differences are usually normal.

The doctor or nurse will measure children's height and weight when they have their checkups. Ask the doctor about each child's growth rate.

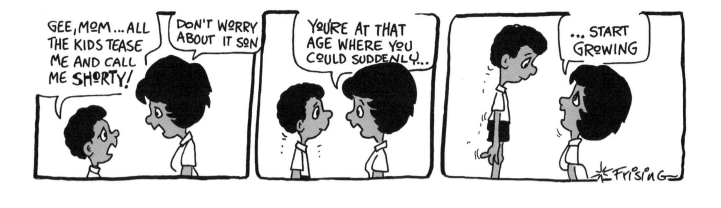

Growth

Children grow at different rates. Some children are tall and some children are short for their age; some are thin and some are stout. Even children in the same family grow at different rates. These differences are usually normal.

Teach children that differences in height and weight are okay. Don't allow them to tease other children about height or weight. It is important that children are happy with their own growth rates.

The doctor or nurse will measure children's height and weight during regular checkups. Ask the doctor about each child's growth rate.

It is important for parents to know their children's heights and weights. For example, when a child is sick, medicine dosage may depend upon age and weight.

If you think a child is overweight, talk with the child's doctor. Do not put a child on a diet unless a doctor says it is necessary. Instead, encourage the child to eat healthy foods. Limit candy, sweets, fried foods, and chips.

Let children run and play outside whenever possible. Healthy food and physical activity help children grow and develop strong bodies.

From *Hip on Health: Health Information for Caregivers and Families* by Charlotte M. Hendricks. Published by Redleaf Press. www.redleafpress.org.

Physical Activity for Infants

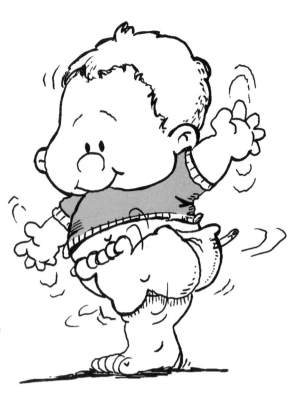

Help infants grow and develop with simple activities together every day:

- Provide lots of tummy time. Place infants on their tummies, allowing them to lift their heads and kick their legs.

- Support infants in standing upright.

- Play games like peekaboo and patty-cake.

- Provide clean, safe floors, and allow infants to explore freely.

From *Hip on Health: Health Information for Caregivers and Families* by Charlotte M. Hendricks. Published by Redleaf Press. www.redleafpress.org.

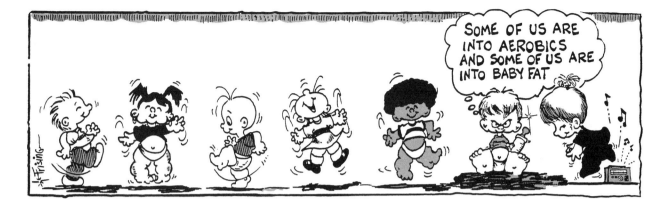

Physical Activity for Infants

You can provide simple activities for infants every day to promote walking, running, reaching, and other skills. Physical activity for infants involves playful interaction.

✓ Provide lots of tummy time while infants are awake. Place them on their tummies, allowing them to lift their heads and kick their legs.

✓ When they can sit up, help them sit between your legs. Place their hands on a ball and roll the ball forward and back.

✓ As they grow, support them in standing upright to help develop balance and strength.

✓ Play games like peekaboo and patty-cake.

✓ Allow infants to explore freely on clean, safe floors. Encourage creeping, crawling, and eventually walking.

✓ Encourage older infants to roll and toss large soft balls.

Avoid infant walkers! Children in walkers can quickly scoot across the floor—often into danger.

Expensive toys are not necessary. Love, gentle caresses, and regular communication are priceless.

From *Hip on Health: Health Information for Caregivers and Families* by Charlotte M. Hendricks. Published by Redleaf Press. www.redleafpress.org.

Toilet Training

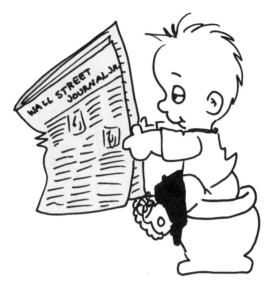

Most children do not become fully toilet trained until they are 2 to 4 years old.

Watch children for signs that they are ready to begin:

- showing discomfort when wearing a dirty diaper

- choosing a particular place to have bowel movements

- showing an interest in or asking questions about the toilet

- wanting to sit on the toilet

- stopping an activity for a few seconds or clutching their diapers

From *Hip on Health: Health Information for Caregivers and Families* by Charlotte M. Hendricks. Published by Redleaf Press. www.redleafpress.org.

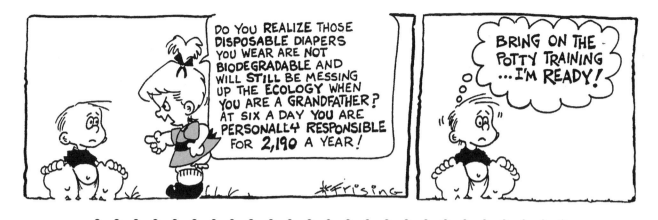

Toilet Training

Toilet training takes a lot of patience. Most children are not fully toilet trained until they are two to four years old. Watch children for signs that they are ready to begin:

- ✓ showing discomfort when wearing dirty diapers

- ✓ choosing a particular area to have bowel movements

- ✓ showing an interest in or asking questions about the toilet

- ✓ wanting to sit on the toilet

There are many ways to teach children to use the toilet. Try several things and see what works best for them. Here are some examples:

- ✓ Show children how you sit on the toilet. Explain what you are doing.

- ✓ Have children sit on the toilet if they wake from their naps with dry diapers. Praise their attempts to use the toilet, even if nothing happens.

- ✓ Do not punish or tease children for mistakes. Toilet training takes time.

- ✓ Children often show that they need to use the toilet. Their faces turn red, they may grunt or squat, or they may stop an activity for a few seconds and clutch their diapers. Put them on the toilet when you see these actions.

- ✓ Dump bowel movement from their diapers into the toilet and let the children flush the toilet.

- ✓ Wash children's hands every time they use the toilet.

Dress children in simple clothes so they can undress themselves quickly. Provide comfortable, toddler-size potty chairs or place toddler-size seats on top of regular toilet seats. Do not flush toilets while children are sitting on them—that can be scary!

From *Hip on Health: Health Information for Caregivers and Families* by Charlotte M. Hendricks. Published by Redleaf Press. www.redleafpress.org.

Weight

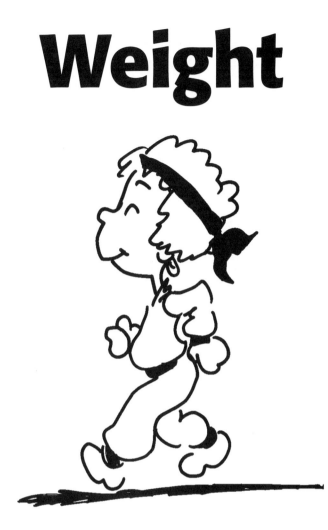

Reduce the risk of childhood weight problems:

- Serve nutritious meals with a variety of foods.

- Limit fried, high-fat, and high-sugar foods.

- Provide healthy snacks.

- Limit TV and screen time.

- Plan physical activities to do with children.

From Hip on Health: Health Information for Caregivers and Families by Charlotte M. Hendricks. Published by Redleaf Press. www.redleafpress.org.

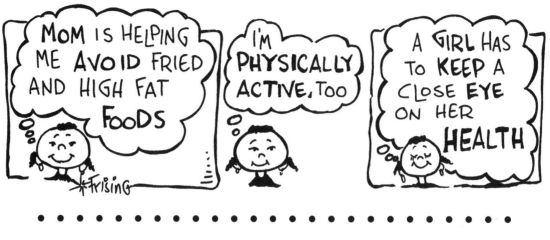

Weight

Many children in the United States are at risk for becoming overweight. High-fat and high-sugar foods and lack of physical activity put children at risk.

Children grow and develop at different rates. Skinny children may be half the size of stout children. Yet both may be very healthy.

Health care providers chart the children's growth, including weight, height, and age. They inform parents of changes and alert them to potential concerns. To promote children's healthy growth and development, provide nutritious foods and encourage daily physical activity.

Adults should provide healthy foods and then let children choose what and how much they want to eat. Help children learn to make healthy decisions by doing the following:

✓ Serve nutritious meals with a variety of foods.

✓ Avoid fried and high-fat foods.

✓ Offer healthy snacks, such as fruit and cheese, instead of candy and cookies

Children need daily physical activity. Limit TV, video games, and other screen time for adults and children alike. Find activities to do together that require moving your bodies. Joining in physical activities with children will help keep you fit too!

From *Hip on Health: Health Information for Caregivers and Families* by Charlotte M. Hendricks. Published by Redleaf Press. www.redleafpress.org.

Allergies

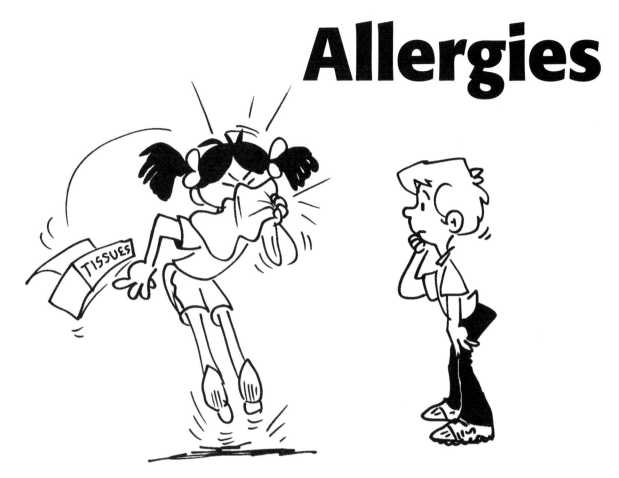

Allergic reactions occur when someone's immune system reacts to a substance. House dust, flower and plant pollen, medicines, foods, cigarette smoke, and insect stings are allergens that may cause reactions.

Talk to a doctor about how to identify and remove possible allergens.

If children have allergies, talk with their doctor about treatment and medicines. Do not use over-the-counter nose sprays or medicines unless the child's doctor says it is okay.

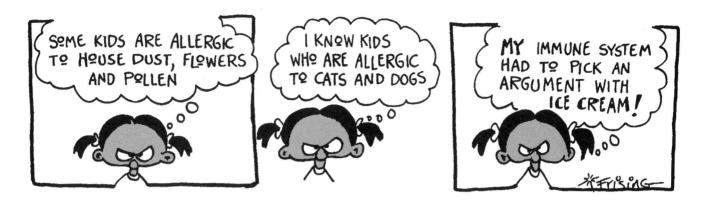

Allergies

Allergic reactions occur when someone's immune system reacts to substances such as house dust, flower and plant pollen, medicines, foods, cigarette smoke, or insect bites. The first time a child is exposed to the substance, such as a certain food, there may be no reaction. However, the immune system may produce antibodies. These antibodies may cause a reaction the next time the child is exposed to the substance.

Allergies produce many symptoms, including sneezing, runny noses, itchy red eyes, and cough. Some allergic reactions can be life threatening. Severe allergic reactions to a food, drug, or insect sting can cause swelling and breathing problems and can be deadly! If you notice that a child has an unusual reaction to any medicine, a bee or other insect sting, or a food, tell the child's doctor. If a child's reaction causes breathing problems, call for emergency help (911) immediately!

A blood or skin test can help identify allergies. Talk to the child's doctor about how to identify and remove possible allergens. If a child does have allergies, talk with the child's doctor about the best treatment and medicines. Do not use over-the-counter nose sprays or medicines unless the child's doctor says it is okay.

Do not smoke or use sprays such as air freshener, hair spray, and perfume around children. Besides triggering allergic reactions, these irritating substances can cause coughing and breathing problems.

From *Hip on Health: Health Information for Caregivers and Families* by Charlotte M. Hendricks. Published by Redleaf Press. www.redleafpress.org.

Asthma

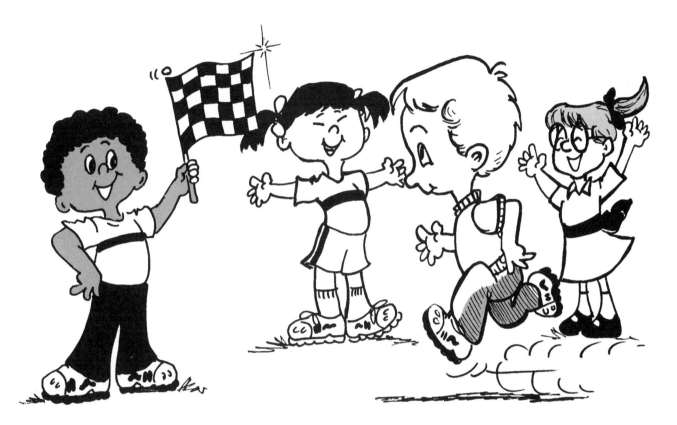

Many children suffer from asthma. Asthma attacks narrow the airway openings and make it hard to breathe.

Colds, allergies, cigarette smoke, perfumes, sprays, and fumes can cause asthma attacks in some children.

Physical activity is important. If children with asthma are not wheezing, they can still run and play. Encourage them to take part in swimming, gymnastics, and other activities.

From *Hip on Health: Health Information for Caregivers and Families* by Charlotte M. Hendricks. Published by Redleaf Press. www.redleafpress.org.

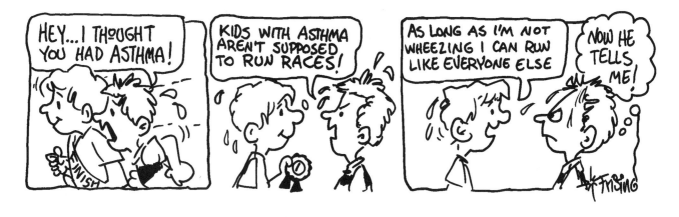

Asthma

A child who often exhibits shortness of breath, coughing, rapid breathing, and wheezing, coughs at night or after running or crying may have asthma. Ask the child's doctor to check for asthma, which is a common condition.

Colds, allergies, cigarette smoke, perfumes, sprays, and fumes can cause asthma attacks. Cold air, physical activity, crying, and yelling can cause hard breathing and may lead to asthma attacks.

During an asthma attack, muscles in the lungs tighten around the airways. The lining inside the airways swells and produces a lot of sticky mucus. This narrows the airway openings and makes breathing more difficult.

Asthma usually can be controlled. Children with asthma should have regular medical checkups. They may need to take certain medicines every day, such as inhalers, liquids, pills, or shots. Some medicines help prevent asthma attacks. Others help during attacks. Never give a child more medicine than the doctor prescribes. Always tell the doctor about any side effects or problems with the medicine. Call the child's doctor anytime you are worried about a child's breathing.

Be sure the child's teacher or caregiver has the correct medicine and phone numbers for you and the child's doctor. Give the teacher a list of substances or activities that can cause asthma attacks, the symptoms the child will have, and what to do. If the child's doctor has written an Asthma Action Plan, give the teacher a copy.

Children with asthma who are not wheezing can run and play with other children. Encourage them to take part in swimming, gymnastics, and other activities.

From *Hip on Health: Health Information for Caregivers and Families* by Charlotte M. Hendricks. Published by Redleaf Press. www.redleafpress.org.

Colds

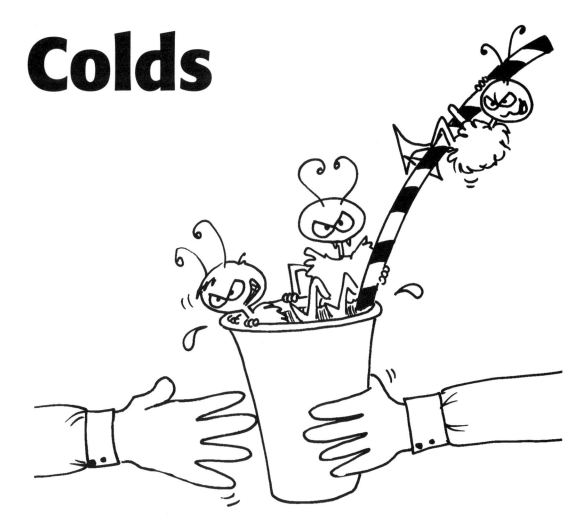

Colds can cause runny noses and sniffles.

Colds are spread by sharing food or drinks with someone who has a cold and by touching someone who has a cold. Cold germs also can be spread by objects, such as toys. Colds are not caused by being outside in cold weather.

Children with colds can go outside if they feel like it.

From *Hip on Health: Health Information for Caregivers and Families* by Charlotte M. Hendricks. Published by Redleaf Press. www.redleafpress.org.

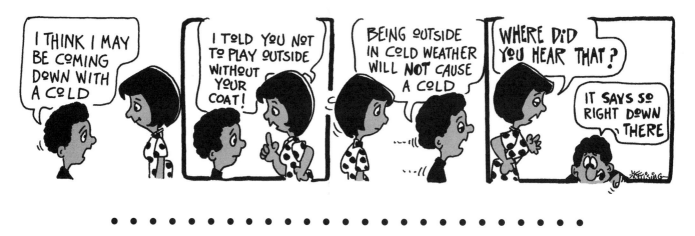

Colds

Colds cause runny noses and sniffles and can make children feel bad.

Respiratory diseases like colds are spread by sharing food or drink with someone who has a cold and by touching someone who has a cold. Cold germs also can be spread by objects, such as toys. Cold germs are also spread through the air. Teach children to cover their mouths and noses when they cough or sneeze.

Colds and flu are caused by viruses. This means antibiotics and other medicines cannot cure them. However, children's doctors may recommend medication such as acetaminophen or ibuprofen to help sick children feel better. Do not give aspirin to children! Cool-mist humidifiers may make breathing easier.

Sometimes colds can lead to sinus infections or ear infections. If a child complains of ear pain or has a fever, call the child's doctor. The child may need an antibiotic.

Do not take children to school or child care if they do not feel well enough to play.

Lots of rest and healthy food help children get well. If they have colds, they can play outside if they feel like it. Being outside in cold weather does not cause colds.

From *Hip on Health: Health Information for Caregivers and Families* by Charlotte M. Hendricks. Published by Redleaf Press. www.redleafpress.org.

Coughs

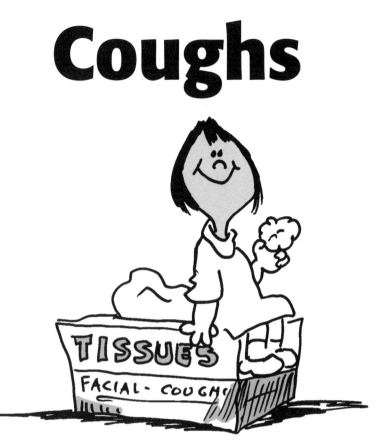

Coughing is a common symptom of childhood illness. Although it can sound awful at times, coughing usually is not a symptom of serious illness. However, in some instances a doctor should be consulted.

Over-the-counter (nonprescription) cough medicine is *not* recommended for young children.

Talk to their doctor or pharmacist before giving any medication to children. Medicines can have dangerous side effects for infants and young children. Never give any medicine that contains alcohol.

From *Hip on Health: Health Information for Caregivers and Families* by Charlotte M. Hendricks. Published by Redleaf Press. www.redleafpress.org.

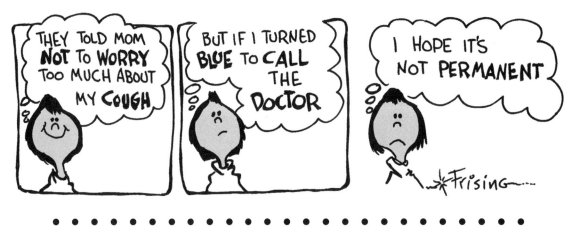

Coughs

Coughing can be a healthy reflex that helps clear airways in the throat and chest, such as when children swallow food or drink the wrong way. This is a good cough.

Coughing is a common symptom of childhood illness. Although it can sound awful at times, it usually is not a symptom of serious illness. However, in some instances a doctor should be consulted. Call a doctor when children experience the following conditions:

✓ difficult breathing

✓ bluish color to the lips, face, or tongue

✓ temperature over 102°F; temperature over 100°F in infants

✓ coughing for over an hour in infants

✓ whooping sound after coughing

✓ noisy, harsh sound when inhaling (breathing in)

✓ wheezing sound when exhaling (breathing out)

✓ "barking" cough

✓ coughing up blood

Talk to children's doctors or a pharmacist before giving any medication. It is helpful to describe the cough when you call.

Over-the-counter (OTC) or nonprescription cough medicine is *not* recommended for young children. Cough medicines can have dangerous side effects in infants and young children.

Never give any OTC medicine that contains alcohol. Alcohol is dangerous for children.

Remember—cough drops are a choking hazard for young children!

From *Hip on Health: Health Information for Caregivers and Families* by Charlotte M. Hendricks. Published by Redleaf Press. www.redleafpress.org.

Croup

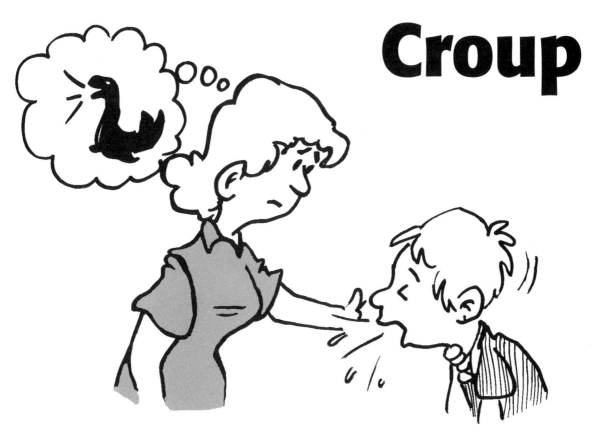

Croup is a respiratory disease caused by a virus. Croup causes a cough that sounds like a seal barking.

Croup can cause children's airways to swell, making it hard for them to breathe. This can be *very serious*.

You should call a doctor *immediately* when children exhibit any of these symptoms:

- cough and cannot stop

- cannot seem to catch their breath

- seem to be getting very tired and cannot stop coughing

From *Hip on Health: Health Information for Caregivers and Families* by Charlotte M. Hendricks. Published by Redleaf Press. www.redleafpress.org.

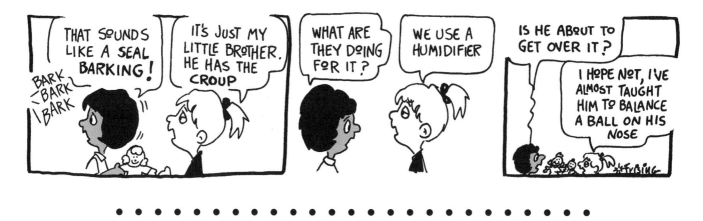

Croup

Croup is a respiratory disease caused by a virus. Croup causes a cough that sounds like a seal barking.

Cool-mist humidifiers may help children with mild croup coughs. Sometimes, children's coughs will stop if you take them outside into cool air or into a bathroom filled with warm steam. Be careful to keep them away from hot water.

Croup can cause inflammation, and swelling and narrowing of the airways. Narrowing makes breathing difficult. This can be *serious*.

Call the child's doctor *immediately* if the child

✓ coughs and cannot stop,

✓ makes a wheezing or odd sound when breathing, especially while inhaling,

✓ cannot seem to get his or her breath, or

✓ seems to be getting tired and cannot stop coughing.

If you are worried about the child's breathing, make the call.

From *Hip on Health: Health Information for Caregivers and Families* by Charlotte M. Hendricks. Published by Redleaf Press. www.redleafpress.org.

Dehydration

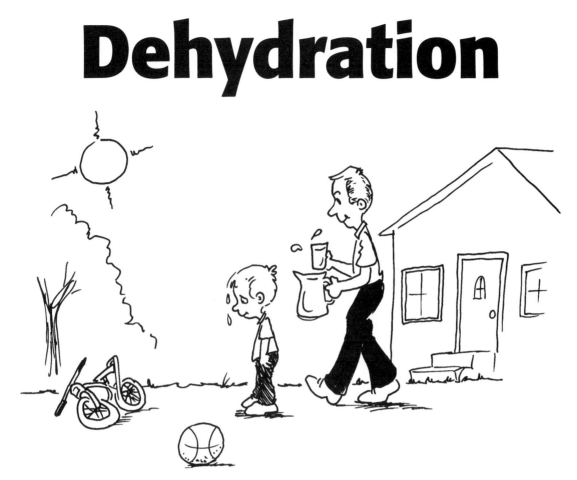

Children normally lose fluids from their bodies when they urinate (pee) or sweat. They lose even more fluid if they vomit or have diarrhea. When they lose too much fluid, they can become *dehydrated*.

Children should drink enough to make them urinate at least every six hours. Dehydrated children may have dry skin and mouth or sunken eyes.

Give children plenty of water and other fluids to drink, especially during hot weather or when they are playing hard.

From *Hip on Health: Health Information for Caregivers and Families* by Charlotte M. Hendricks. Published by Redleaf Press. www.redleafpress.org.

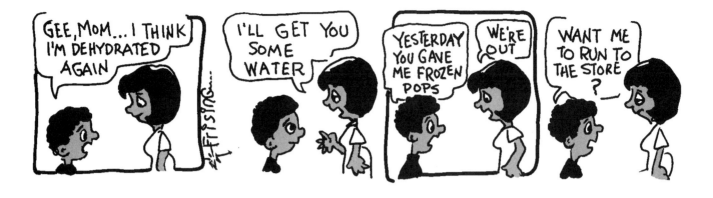

Dehydration

Children normally lose fluid from their bodies when they perspire (sweat) and urinate (pee). They perspire more when they play outside in warm or hot weather or wear too much clothing. They lose fluid when they vomit or have diarrhea. When they lose too much fluid, they can become dehydrated. Dehydration can be serious, especially for infants and young children.

Thirst is *not* a reliable sign of dehydration. Children can be satisfied by a few sips of water and still be dehydrated. They should drink enough to make them urinate at least every six hours. Children who are dehydrated may not urinate this often and may have dry skin and mouth or sunken eyes. Watch children carefully for signs of dehydration.

Children who have vomited or who have diarrhea should be given small sips of clear liquids to replace the fluids lost. It is usually best to give water or clear fluids, such as caffeine-free flavored waters, gelatins, and frozen pops. Ask the child's doctor or pharmacist about liquids such as sports drinks. Call a doctor if you think a child is becoming dehydrated or if vomiting or diarrhea lasts more than one day.

From *Hip on Health: Health Information for Caregivers and Families* by Charlotte M. Hendricks. Published by Redleaf Press. www.redleafpress.org.

Dermatitis

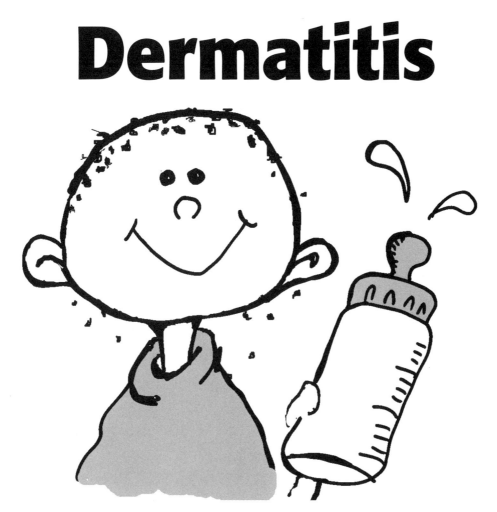

Seborrheic dermatitis, better known as cradle cap, commonly occurs in infants.

Cradle cap appears as thick white or yellow scales on the scalp. Some children have only a small patch of scales, while others have scales all over their heads.

Cradle cap is not contagious and usually clears within a few months. Contact a doctor if it does not clear, seems severe, or spreads to children's faces or bodies.

From *Hip on Health: Health Information for Caregivers and Families* by Charlotte M. Hendricks. Published by Redleaf Press. www.redleafpress.org.

105

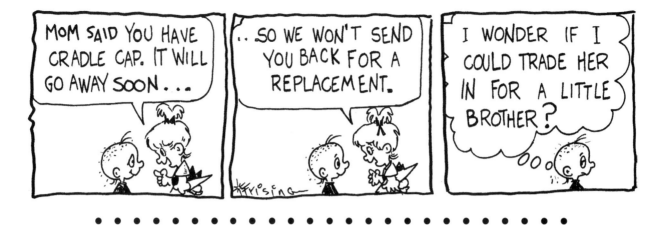

Dermatitis

Dermatitis is a general term used to describe a variety of skin inflammations. **Cradle cap** is a dermatitis that commonly occurs in infants.

Cradle cap appears as thick white or yellow scales on the scalp. Some children have only a small patch of scales, while others have scales all over their heads. This dermatitis can even occur on the eyebrows, eyelids, ears, crease of the nose, back of the neck, diaper area, or armpits. Cradle cap may cause mild itching.

Cradle cap is not contagious and usually clears within a few months. Washing children's scalps daily with mild shampoo can help loosen and remove the cradle cap scales. Contact a doctor if the condition does not clear, seems severe, or spreads to children's faces or bodies.

Eczema, another type of dermatitis, is an itchy inflammation of the skin. Its symptoms vary. Eczema may cause dry, itchy red skin with small bumps. It can also cause red, crusted, or open lesions on the skin. Rashes may become worse if children rub and scratch their skin.

In infants, rashes usually start on the face or over elbows and knees. In older children, rashes usually appear on the arms, inside the elbows, and behind the knees. They may spread to other areas of the body.

Eczema is not contagious. Contact a doctor if you suspect children have eczema, or if they have any unexplained rashes.

Eczema may flare occasionally and then go away. Here are some ways to help avoid flare-ups and reduce the discomfort:

✓ Give cool baths or showers; avoid hot water. Always supervise children closely!

✓ Use mild unscented soap or body wash.

✓ Pat skin dry after bathing. Do not scrub or rub with toweling.

✓ Dress children in soft, lightweight clothes, like cotton ones.

Diarrhea

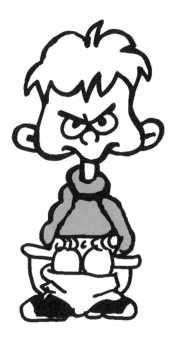

Diarrhea can occur when children's bodies react to something, such as antibiotics or other medicines. Allergies to food, such as milk, can also cause diarrhea.

Infectious diarrhea is caused by germs. The best way to prevent it is to wash hands often with soap and running water. Help children wash their hands after toileting, playing outside, and before eating.

From *Hip on Health: Health Information for Caregivers and Families* by Charlotte M. Hendricks. Published by Redleaf Press. www.redleafpress.org.

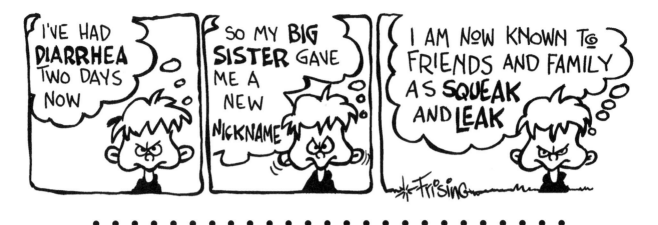

Diarrhea

Diarrhea can occur when children's bodies react to something, such as antibiotics or other medicines. Sorbitol, a sugar found in some liquid medicines and in foods such as apple juice and some fruit drinks, can cause diarrhea in young children. Allergies to food, such as milk, also can cause diarrhea.

Diarrhea caused by germs is called infectious diarrhea and can be spread to others. Some infectious diarrheas—for example, those caused by rotavirus, salmonella bacteria, and the parasite giardia—can be more serious.

Rotavirus disease is easily spread among young children. It usually begins with fever, nausea, and vomiting, followed by severe diarrhea. Diarrhea may last up to nine days. Rotavirus is preventable through immunization.

Salmonella bacteria can be found in foods containing raw or undercooked eggs, poultry, or meat. Salmonella can also be found on pet turtles, reptiles, and baby chicks. Make children wash their hands immediately after handling these to prevent infection.

Giardia is a parasite. It easily spreads among young children, who may not always wash their hands well after toileting. Children also can get giardia by drinking contaminated water or by swallowing water in swimming or wading pools.

The best way to prevent infectious diarrhea is to wash hands often with soap and running water, especially after using the toilet and before handling food.

Diarrhea can cause dehydration, especially in infants and young children. If children cannot keep fluids down and have dry skin, sunken eyes, or are not urinating at least every six hours, call their doctor. If they continue to have diarrhea for several hours, or if you are worried, call a doctor.

Ear Infection

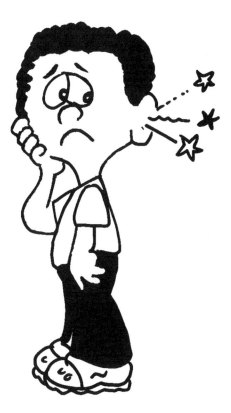

Ear infections can be caused by bacteria in the canal that connects the ear with the back of the nose. This often happens when children have colds or other respiratory infections.

They may develop pain and fever, red or itchy ears, or fluid coming from the ears. Ear infections can affect their hearing.

Call their doctors if you think they have ear infections.

From *Hip on Health: Health Information for Caregivers and Families* by Charlotte M. Hendricks. Published by Redleaf Press. www.redleafpress.org.

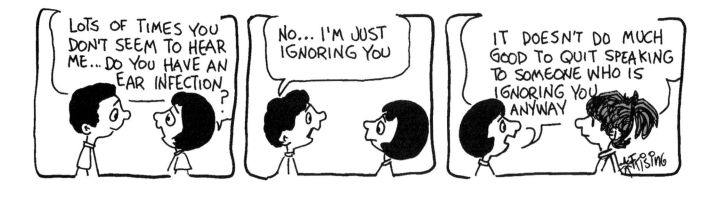

Ear Infection

Do children hear you? Children who do not respond to you may have a hearing problem. Ask their doctor about hearing testing.

Hearing problems can be caused by ear infections, water in the ear, or damage to the eardrums. You can prevent permanent hearing loss by getting early and proper treatment for children with hearing problems.

Young children often get ear infections, especially if they have colds or upper respiratory infections. Ear infections can be caused by bacteria in the canal that connects the ear with the nose. Children may have pain and fever, red or itchy ears, and fluid coming from the ears.

Most ear infections are caused by pneumococcal bacteria. Many ear infections can be prevented by immunization against these bacteria.

Doctors may recommend ear tubes for children with frequent ear infections. These tiny tubes are placed in the eardrum and create little openings to allow air into the middle ear, help it heal, and stop infections.

Ear tubes are inserted by a surgeon. Children cannot feel the tubes after they are in place. Ear tubes usually stay in place for twelve to eighteen months. The tubes usually come out by themselves.

From *Hip on Health: Health Information for Caregivers and Families* by Charlotte M. Hendricks. Published by Redleaf Press. www.redleafpress.org.

Fever

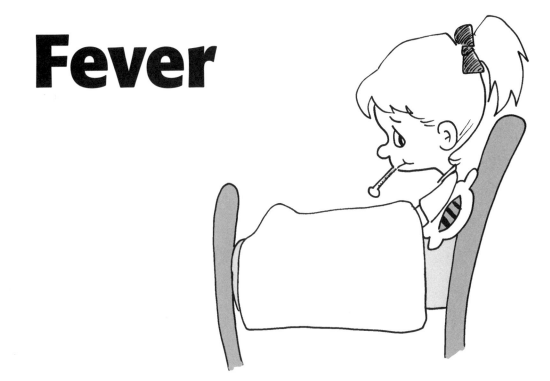

Children can run high fevers when they are sick. Call a doctor *immediately* when infants under one year old run temperatures of 100°F or higher.

Call children's doctors immediately when fever and other symptoms like these occur:

- The child faints or has convulsions.

- The child seems confused or cannot be calmed down.

- The child is unusually quiet or sleepy, has a hard time breathing, has a stiff neck, has a rash, or is vomiting.

- The child is not drinking fluids.

From *Hip on Health: Health Information for Caregivers and Families* by Charlotte M. Hendricks. Published by Redleaf Press. www.redleafpress.org.

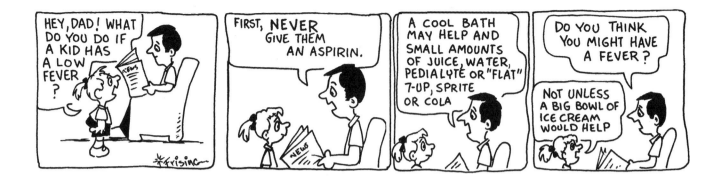

Fever

Children can run high fevers very quickly. Do you know how to take a child's temperature? Do you have a thermometer?

A plastic digital thermometer that beeps is fast, safe, and easy to use. A safe way to take children's temperatures is to place the bulb of the thermometer high in their armpits. Make sure the armpit is dry and there is no clothing between the skin and the thermometer. Hold the child's arm snugly against the body.

For older infants and children, temperature can be measured using a tympanic (ear) thermometer or a temporal artery (forehead) thermometer. Follow the manufacturer's instructions for these thermometers.

A temperature of over 100°F is considered fever. Although fevers are not usually dangerous, you should call the doctor when a temperature is over 101°F or the fever lasts more than thirty-six hours.

Call the child's doctor *immediately* if any of these symptoms occur along with fever:

✓ The child is under one year old and has a temperature of 100°F or higher.

✓ The child faints or has convulsions.

✓ The child seems confused, disoriented, or cannot be calmed down.

✓ The child is unusually quiet or sleepy, has a hard time breathing, has a stiff neck, has a rash, is vomiting, or just acts sick.

✓ The child is not drinking fluids.

Call the doctor immediately if a child who has sickle-cell anemia or other chronic condition has fever. It could indicate a more serious infection.

From *Hip on Health: Health Information for Caregivers and Families* by Charlotte M. Hendricks. Published by Redleaf Press. www.redleafpress.org.

Food Allergies

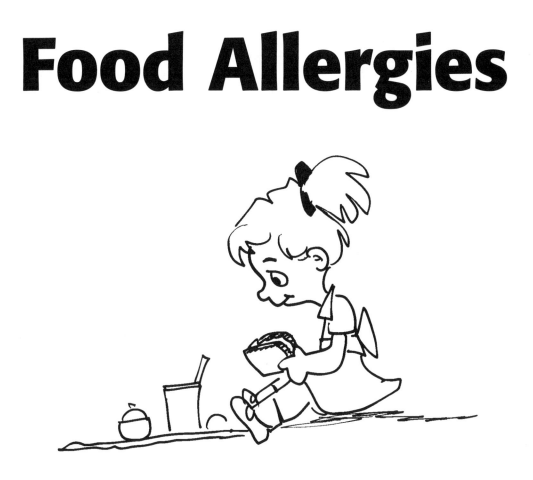

If children feel bad or have physical symptoms after eating certain foods, then they may have allergies or intolerance to specific foods or food additives.

Foods that commonly cause allergic reactions include milk, eggs, peanuts, wheat, soy, fish, shellfish, and tree nuts.

Allergic reactions can be mild, such as headache or a rash. Severe reactions can cause swelling of the tongue and throat, breathing difficulties, or loss of consciousness. If any of these occur, call 911!

From *Hip on Health: Health Information for Caregivers and Families* by Charlotte M. Hendricks. Published by Redleaf Press. www.redleafpress.org.

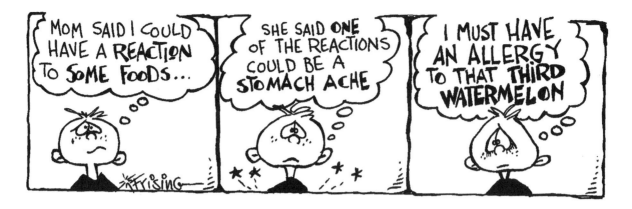

Food Allergies

If children seem to feel bad or have physical symptoms after eating certain foods, then they may have allergies or intolerance to specific foods or food additives. Here are some examples:

✓ Milk sugar (lactose) intolerance can cause stomachaches.

✓ Chemicals in cheese and chocolate, preservatives, and food dyes can cause headaches.

Some children are allergic to certain foods or additives. Foods that commonly cause allergic reactions include milk, eggs, peanuts, wheat, soy, fish, shellfish, and tree nuts. Foods can cause reactions whether they are eaten raw or cooked. Symptoms may occur after eating even tiny amounts of the food.

Reactions can be mild, such as headache, diarrhea, or hives (red, itchy, swollen areas of the skin).

Severe reactions can cause swelling of the tongue and throat, breathing difficulty, and loss of consciousness. If children develop breathing difficulties or become unconscious, call emergency help immediately!

Talk to the children's doctors if you think food is causing physical reactions. The doctor can help you identify the food or additive. The first treatment is to avoid the foods that cause problems.

Some foods or additives have several different names. Learn the technical or scientific names for foods and read food labels carefully. Ask about ingredients when eating out. Be sure all adults who care for children with food allergies avoid serving these foods.

From *Hip on Health: Health Information for Caregivers and Families* by Charlotte M. Hendricks. Published by Redleaf Press. www.redleafpress.org.

Head Lice

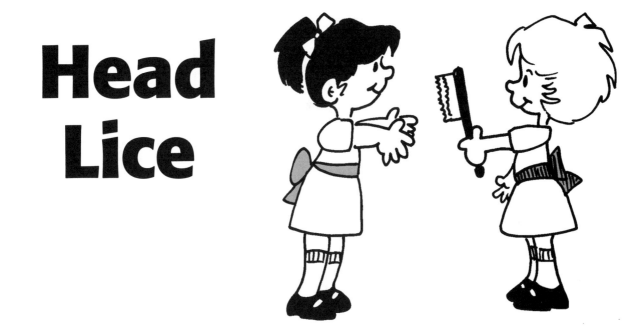

Head lice are small insects that live on people's scalps and lay their eggs (nits) on the hair. Lice can cause itching and pain. Scratching can cause skin infections.

Anyone can get lice. You can get lice from another person if your hair touches their hair, if you share hats or hair brushes, or if your clothes touch.

Do the following to get rid of head lice:

- Ask a pharmacist about special shampoos to kill lice and their eggs.

- Use a special comb to remove nits from hair.

- Wash clothes, blankets, and toys in hot water.

- Vacuum rugs and floors.

From *Hip on Health: Health Information for Caregivers and Families* by Charlotte M. Hendricks. Published by Redleaf Press. www.redleafpress.org.

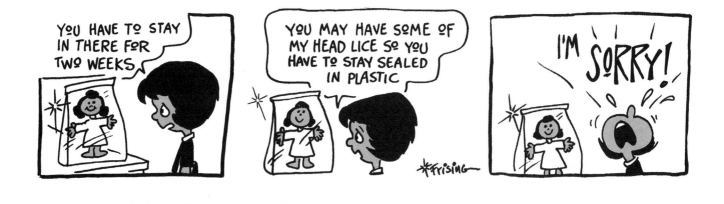

Head Lice

Head lice live only on people—not on animals. These small insects can be spread by direct head-to-head contact or by sharing objects such as hats, combs, pillows, or headphones.

Children may not show early signs of head lice. Later, they may scratch their head, be irritable, or have red patches on their scalps or necks. Scratching can cause skin conditions like impetigo.

Head lice are usually dark tan, brown, or black and are very small (almost as small as this dot ·). Look for yellow, silver, or light brown nits (eggs) attached to the hair near the scalp. Nits are very hard to pull off the hair.

If a child has lice, the entire family should be checked for lice. Call the child's doctor, the health department, or a pharmacist, and ask about special shampoos for head lice. Check with a doctor about treatments for infants or women who are pregnant or nursing. Nits should be removed by using a special comb.

Lice and nits can live on clothing, beds, or other items. Soak all washable items in hot water for ten minutes. Wash clothing, sheets, and towels in hot water and dry in a hot dryer for at least twenty minutes.

Place nonwashable items, such as stuffed toys, in a tightly sealed plastic bag for two weeks. Then open the bag outdoors and shake the toys thoroughly.

Vacuum carpets and furniture carefully for several days to remove lice and nits. Anti-lice sprays are not recommended because children can breathe in the fumes.

From *Hip on Health: Health Information for Caregivers and Families* by Charlotte M. Hendricks. Published by Redleaf Press. www.redleafpress.org.

Impetigo

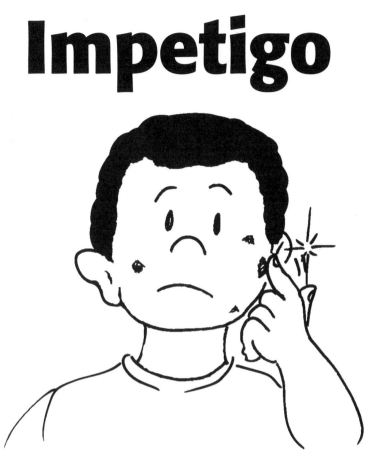

Impetigo is an infection of the skin. It starts as reddened areas that become pus-filled blisters.

Sores usually occur on the face, hands, and legs but can appear anywhere on the body.

Children can get impetigo from other people who have it. They can also get impetigo by scratching insect bites or itchy rashes, such as those caused by poison ivy.

Impetigo may not go away by itself. It is usually treated with an antibiotic ointment and sometimes an oral antibiotic.

From *Hip on Health: Health Information for Caregivers and Families* by Charlotte M. Hendricks. Published by Redleaf Press. www.redleafpress.org.

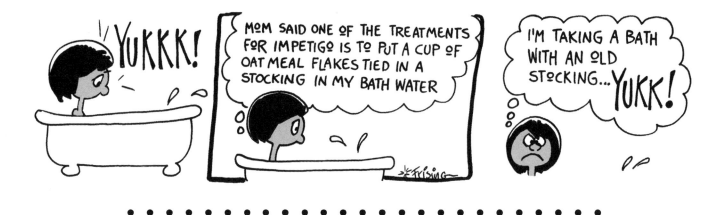

Impetigo

Impetigo is an infection of the skin. It starts as reddened areas that become pus-filled blisters. The blisters easily break and form thick brownish scabs. Sores usually occur on the face, hands, and legs, but can appear anywhere on the body.

Children can get impetigo from other people who have it. They can also get impetigo by scratching insect bites or itchy rashes, such as those caused by poison ivy. Impetigo bacteria may be found under children's fingernails, and when children scratch and break the skin, the bacteria can infect their skin.

Impetigo may not go away by itself and is commonly treated with an antibiotic. Children with impetigo should be treated in the following ways:

✓ Wash the sores two to three times each day with soap and water. Give a bath or shower each day.

✓ Wash children's hands and your hands often with soap and water. Use separate towels, washcloths, sheets, combs, and other items for children with impetigo.

✓ If a doctor or pharmacist has suggested an antibiotic ointment, apply it as directed.

✓ If a doctor has prescribed an oral antibiotic (pills or liquid), be sure to give the medicine as directed until all of it is gone.

✓ Do not allow children to return to school until they have been taking the prescribed medicine for at least twenty-four hours.

✓ If the sores itch, bathe children in lukewarm water with either ½ cup of baking soda or 1 cup of oatmeal flakes tied in a stocking or net bag. Mix this into the bath water.

From *Hip on Health: Health Information for Caregivers and Families* by Charlotte M. Hendricks. Published by Redleaf Press. www.redleafpress.org.

Nosebleed

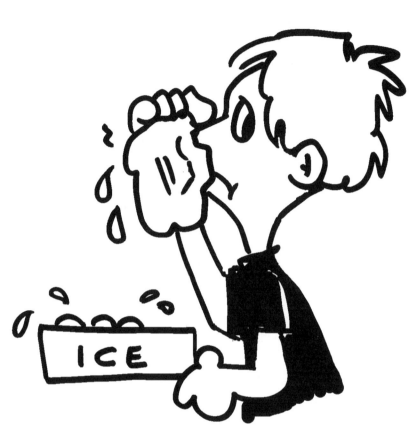

Children may get nosebleeds if they bump their noses, pick them, sneeze, or blow their noses hard.

You can usually stop a nosebleed by tilting the head forward and gently holding the nostrils closed. A cold, wet cloth or ice pack against the nose may help.

Nosebleeds usually are not serious.

From *Hip on Health: Health Information for Caregivers and Families* by Charlotte M. Hendricks. Published by Redleaf Press. www.redleafpress.org.

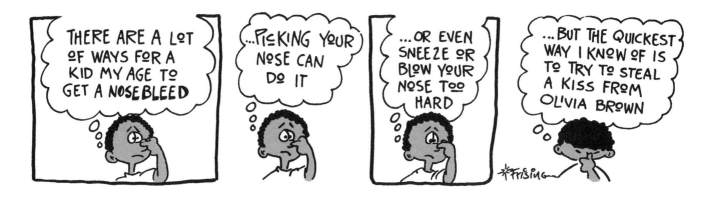

Nosebleed

Children get nosebleeds if they bump or pick their noses, sneeze, or blow their noses hard. Some children get nosebleeds very easily. Nosebleeds can be frightening for them. Calm them, and let them know that the bleeding will stop soon.

Here are ways to stop the bleeding:

✓ Help children sit up with heads tilted slightly forward.

✓ Pinch the nostrils closed. Apply gentle pressure for at least five minutes. Apply a cloth-wrapped cold pack to children's noses and cheeks while applying pressure.

✓ Gently release their noses. If bleeding starts again, reapply the pressure for ten minutes this time.

After the nosebleed stops, gently clean any blood from the child's face and skin. Discourage children from blowing or picking the nose.

Call their doctor if the nosebleed cannot easily be controlled after fifteen minutes, is accompanied by dizziness or weakness, or occurs after a blow to the head or a fall.

Talk to children about the importance of not touching someone else's blood. Blood can contain disease-causing germs, including those that cause hepatitis or HIV infection.

Pinkeye

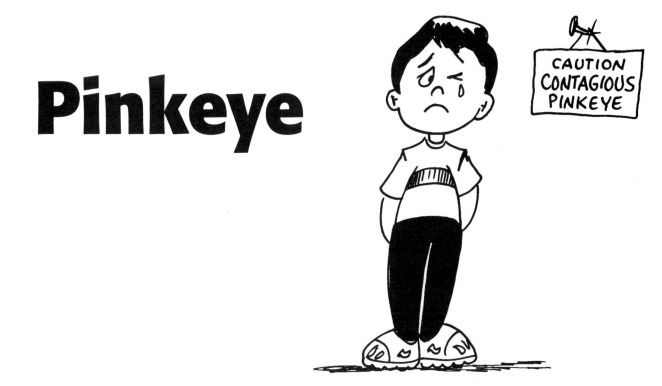

Pinkeye (conjunctivitis) can be caused by viruses or bacteria. It can be very contagious!

Either one or both eyes may have any of these symptoms:

- Eye is red and sensitive to light.

- Eyelid is slightly swollen.

- Eye has a thick discharge that becomes crusty.

- Eye is itchy or watery.

Ask children's doctors about medicine for pinkeye. Do not use over-the-counter eyedrops unless the doctor recommends it.

From *Hip on Health: Health Information for Caregivers and Families* by Charlotte M. Hendricks. Published by Redleaf Press. www.redleafpress.org.

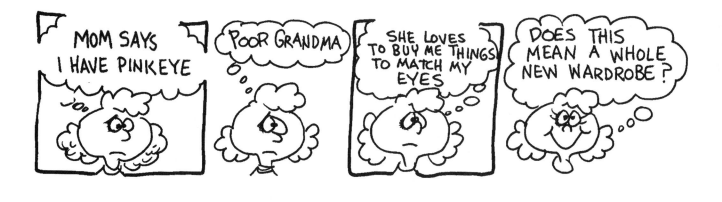

Pinkeye

Pinkeye (conjunctivitis) can be caused by viruses or bacteria. It can be very contagious.

When children with pinkeye touch their eyes, the germs get transferred to their hands. If they then touch another child or a toy, they spread the germs. Pinkeye can also be spread through tissues, washcloths, or towels. Wash your hands carefully before and after helping children with pinkeye.

Either one or both eyes may have any of these symptoms:

- ✓ Eyeball or inner lining of the eyelid is red.
- ✓ Light hurts the eyes.
- ✓ Eyelid is slightly swollen.
- ✓ Eye has a thick discharge.
- ✓ Eyelid has dried crust and is hard to open after sleeping.
- ✓ Eye is itchy.
- ✓ Eye is watery or teary.

When children have pinkeye and their eyelids become very swollen, or the skin around the eye and cheeks become swollen, warm, or red, call the doctor immediately. The infection can be very serious.

Ask children's doctors about medicine for pinkeye. Do not use over-the-counter eyedrops unless the doctor recommends it.

From *Hip on Health: Health Information for Caregivers and Families* by Charlotte M. Hendricks. Published by Redleaf Press. www.redleafpress.org.

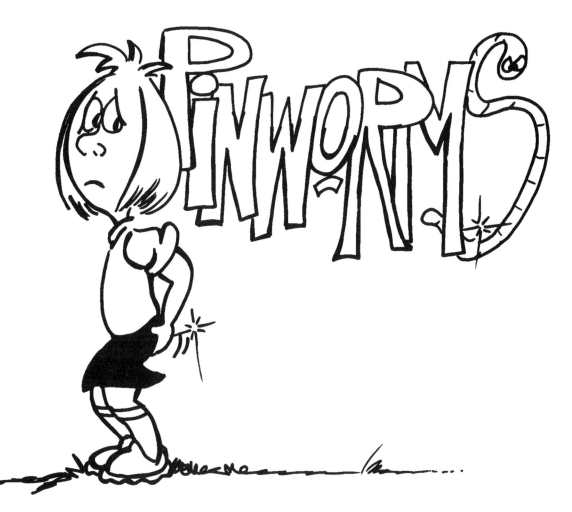

Pinworms are white, very thin worms about ¼ to ½ inch long. They can cause itching around a child's anus (bottom).

When children have a pinworm infection, all their family members may need to take medicine. Ask a doctor or pharmacist about medicines that can be purchased without a prescription.

Help prevent pinworm infection. Teach children to scrub their hands and fingernails completely before eating and after using the toilet.

From *Hip on Health: Health Information for Caregivers and Families* by Charlotte M. Hendricks. Published by Redleaf Press. www.redleafpress.org.

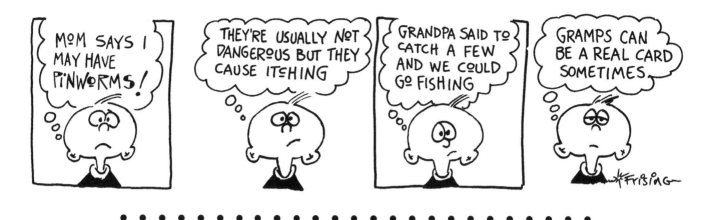

Pinworms

Pinworms are white, very thin worms about ¼–½ inch long. They do not usually cause serious health problems, but they can cause itching around a child's anus (bottom). Scratching can then irritate the area. When children scratch, pinworm eggs can get under the fingernails and be passed to others by direct contact or through shared toys, clothing, and bedding.

If you think children may have a pinworm infection, use a flashlight to check their bottoms a few hours after they go to bed or early in the morning. Look for tiny, white, threadlike worms that move. Do this for two nights in a row. If you do not see pinworms and the children still itch, ask their doctor to check for pinworm eggs.

When children have pinworms, all their family members may need to take medicine. Ask their doctor or pharmacist about medicine that is available without a prescription. There are also medicines that a doctor can prescribe. The medicine will get rid of the pinworms but not the unhatched eggs. A second dose of medicine is needed two weeks later to get rid of pinworms that have hatched since the first treatment. The medicine should stop the itching in about a week. If children still itch or the skin around the anus becomes red or sore, call the children's doctors.

The following actions will help prevent children from getting a pinworm infection:

✓ Help children scrub hands and fingernails completely before eating and after using the toilet.

✓ Vacuum or wet mop children's entire room once a week. This removes pinworm eggs scattered on the floor.

✓ Wash clothes and bed sheets in hot water to kill pinworm eggs.

Rashes

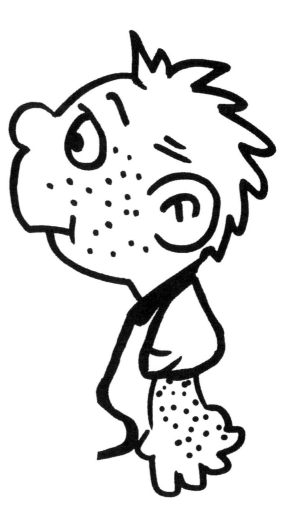

Most skin rashes are not dangerous. Allergic reactions can cause skin rash, as can illness like roseola, fifth disease, strep, measles, and chicken pox.

Rashes can be symptoms of more serious disorders, such as Lyme disease or Rocky Mountain spotted fever, which are diseases spread through tick bites.

Check with a doctor when children have unexplained rashes.

From *Hip on Health: Health Information for Caregivers and Families* by Charlotte M. Hendricks. Published by Redleaf Press. www.redleafpress.org.

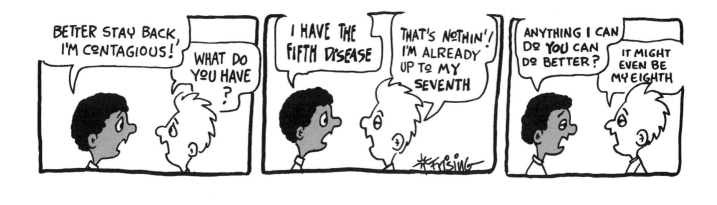

Rashes

Skin rashes can be caused by illnesses or allergic reactions. Most are not dangerous.

Fifth disease is a rash caused by a parvovirus. It is contagious but usually is not serious. For most children, the only symptom is a light red rash beginning on the cheeks and face. The rash can spread to the backs of the arms and legs or all over the body. It may fade some and then reappear and may look worse when the children become hot. The rash is usually gone in about five days, but it may reappear occasionally for several weeks.

This rash may cause children to be uncomfortable and irritable. Be patient with them. Lots of rest will help them feel better. If they seem very uncomfortable or start having other symptoms, such as fever, call a doctor.

Roseola is also caused by a virus. Children with roseola may have high fever for several days and are contagious during this time. After the fever breaks, distinctive, pinkish-red rashes develop on their trunks. The rash may spread to the neck, face, arms, and legs.

Roseola is common among infants and young children. It usually gets better in about a week.

Other diseases, such as measles and chicken pox, also cause rashes. Prevent these diseases by having children immunized.

Rashes may be symptoms of more serious diseases, such as Lyme disease or Rocky Mountain spotted fever. These diseases spread through tick bites.

Check with children's doctors when children have unexplained rashes.

From *Hip on Health: Health Information for Caregivers and Families* by Charlotte M. Hendricks. Published by Redleaf Press. www.redleafpress.org.

Scabies

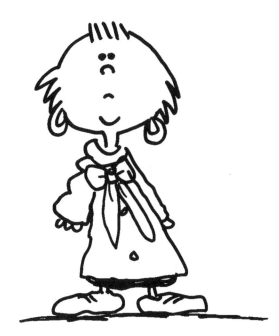

Scabies is a skin infection caused by tiny mites. Anyone can get scabies by sharing clothing or prolonged close contact with an infected person.

To get rid of children's scabies, ask a doctor about prescribed cream or lotion to kill the mites and their eggs.

Wash clothes, towels, blankets, and toys in hot soapy water. Vacuum carpets and mop floors for several days.

From *Hip on Health: Health Information for Caregivers and Families* by Charlotte M. Hendricks. Published by Redleaf Press. www.redleafpress.org.

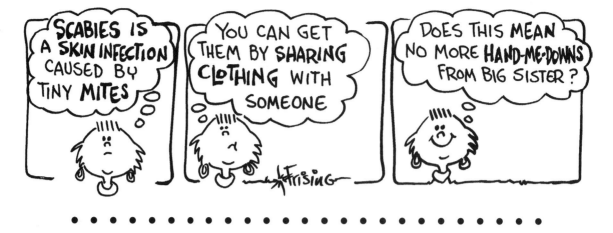

Scabies

Scabies is a skin infection caused by tiny mites. Anyone can get scabies. They are spread from person to person by prolonged close contact, such as sharing the same bed, clothing, or towels. Children do not get scabies from animals.

The microscopic mites burrow into the top layer of skin to lay eggs, which may cause a rash and intense itching.

The infection begins as small itchy blisters that break when a child scratches them. Arms and hands are most often affected, especially between the fingers, the inner part of the wrists, and under the arms. When children scratch these areas, they may develop other skin infections, such as impetigo.

If children develop scabies, the doctor may recommend that their families be treated. Ointment, cream, or lotion may be prescribed for rubbing over the entire body from the neck down. A second treatment one week later may be recommended.

Do not use this medicine on infants! Women who are pregnant or nursing also should not use this medicine. Talk to a doctor—be sure you have the correct medicine and know how to use it.

Mites can live for two to three days in clothing, bedding, or dust. Wash clothes, towels, bed sheets and blankets, and toys in hot soapy water. Vacuum carpets and mop floors carefully for several days.

From *Hip on Health: Health Information for Caregivers and Families* by Charlotte M. Hendricks. Published by Redleaf Press. www.redleafpress.org.

Sore Throat

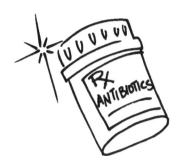

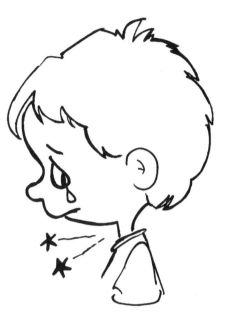

Sore throats may be caused by strep bacteria. These usually cause very sore throats and fevers and may also cause stomachaches, rashes, or general sick feelings. Children's doctors can test for strep throat. It must be treated with antibiotics for a specified period of time, such as 7 to 10 days.

Children may feel better after taking medicine for two or three days, but the medicine should be continued until all of it is gone.

If strep throat is not cured, it can lead to more serious diseases. Taking all the medicine is the only way to cure strep throat.

From *Hip on Health: Health Information for Caregivers and Families* by Charlotte M. Hendricks. Published by Redleaf Press. www.redleafpress.org.

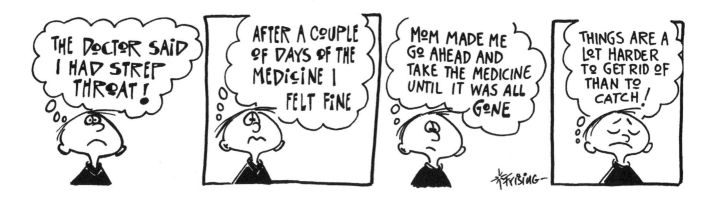

Sore Throat

Sore throat is a common complaint among children. Sore throats may be caused by viruses or bacteria. Dry air, talking, and shouting can also cause dry, irritated throats.

Pain from sore throats may be decreased by using cool-mist humidifiers in rooms where children sleep. Their doctor may suggest pain relievers, such as acetaminophen or ibuprofen. Older children can gargle with warm salt water (1 teaspoon of salt in 1 cup warm of water).

Strep throat is caused by a bacterial infection. It usually causes a very sore throat and fever and may include stomachache, headache, rash, or a general sick feeling. Children's doctors can test for strep throat. It must be treated with antibiotics for a specified period of time, usually seven to ten days. Children may feel better after taking medicine for two or three days, but the medicine should be continued until all of it is gone.

If strep throat is not treated with the correct medicine for the specified period of time, it can lead to more serious diseases, such as rheumatic fever, heart problems, and kidney disorders.

From *Hip on Health: Health Information for Caregivers and Families* by Charlotte M. Hendricks. Published by Redleaf Press. www.redleafpress.org.

Thrush

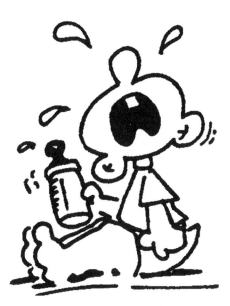

Thrush is caused by a yeast infection. It is very common in infants.

Thrush causes creamy white patches on the lining of and around infants' mouths. These sores can be painful and may bleed slightly if rubbed.

Thrush usually clears up without any treatment within a week or two. If it does not clear up, or if infants are having pain or trouble feeding, contact a doctor. The doctor may prescribe medication to clear the infection. If infants have trouble eating because of pain, the doctor may also recommend a pain medication.

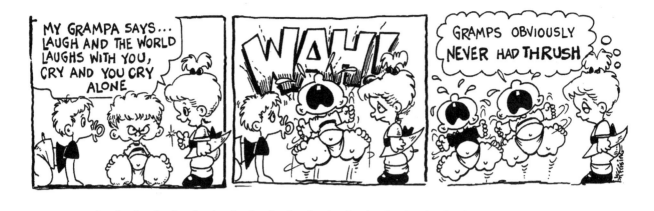

Thrush

Thrush is caused by the fungus *Candida albicans.* Candida, a yeast, is normally found in the mouth and is usually harmless. But sometimes the fungus grows too much, builds up on the lining of the mouth, and causes thrush. It is hard to know what triggers thrush. Sometimes it occurs when an infant takes antibiotics for a bacterial infection. It can also occur if a breast-feeding mother takes antibiotics. Antibiotics can kill off the bacteria that normally keep Candida from growing.

Thrush is a very common infection in infants. Breast-feeding infants and mothers can pass the infection back and forth.

Thrush causes creamy white patches on the lining of and around infants' mouths. These sores can be painful and may bleed slightly if rubbed. Sometimes, thrush spreads to the roof of the mouth, the gums, and the back of the throat.

Infants with thrush may have trouble feeding and may start crying while nursing or sucking on bottles or pacifiers. They may be fussy and irritable.

Thrush usually clears up without any treatment within a week or two. If it does not clear up, or infants have pain or trouble feeding, contact a doctor. The doctor may prescribe medication to clear the infection. If pain is keeping infants from eating, a doctor may recommend a pain medication.

Sometimes infants with thrush also develop a yeast diaper infection. If that happens, a doctor can prescribe antifungal medication to use in the diaper area.

From *Hip on Health: Health Information for Caregivers and Families* by Charlotte M. Hendricks. Published by Redleaf Press. www.redleafpress.org.

Tinea

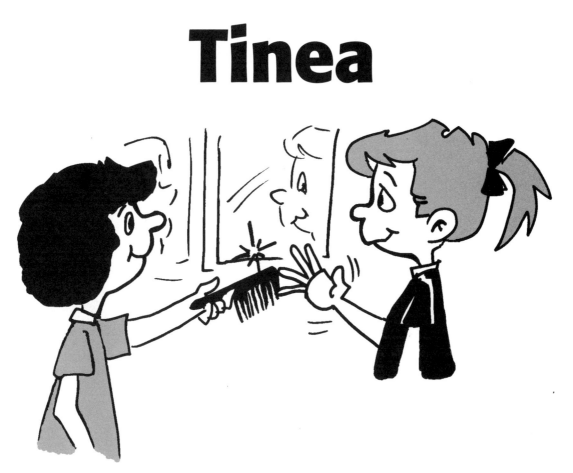

Tinea (ringworm) is a fungal infection that usually affects scalps, trunks, or feet.

Tinea starts as small red bumps that spread outward, leaving red, scaly outer rings. These sores may itch.

Tinea is spread by touching someone who has the sores. Children can also get it by sharing hats, combs, or towels with infected people.

If children contract tinea, ask their doctor or pharmacist about medicine to treat it.

From *Hip on Health: Health Information for Caregivers and Families* by Charlotte M. Hendricks. Published by Redleaf Press. www.redleafpress.org.

133

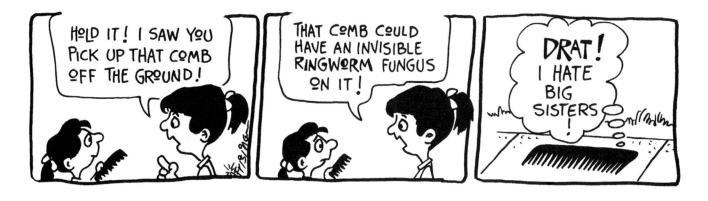

Tinea

Ringworm and athlete's foot are types of skin infection caused by a fungus. These infections are known as *tinea*.

Ringworm usually affects the scalp, trunk, or feet. Ringworm of the scalp may start as a small sore that resembles a pimple. It may look like dandruff and can cause some hair to fall out or break off. It can cause the scalp to become swollen, tender, and red.

Ringworm elsewhere on the body starts as small red bumps that spread outward. The centers clear, leaving red, scaly outer rings. These sores may itch. Ringworm does not produce scabs, pus, or crusts.

Athlete's foot usually affects the soles of the feet and the spaces between toes. It causes a scaly rash that usually itches and burns.

Ringworm and athlete's foot are contagious. The fungus is spread by direct contact (touching the rash of an infected person) and by sharing contaminated objects, such as hats, combs and brushes, and towels, with an infected person. Teach children to avoid sharing these items and to avoid walking barefoot in public areas like locker rooms and shared shower areas.

Cover sores with bandages and wear socks and shoes to prevent scratching and spreading the disease.

Tinea can often be treated with over-the-counter (nonprescription) medicines. If the sores do not get better after a week of treatment, call the children's doctors.

From *Hip on Health: Health Information for Caregivers and Families* by Charlotte M. Hendricks. Published by Redleaf Press. www.redleafpress.org.

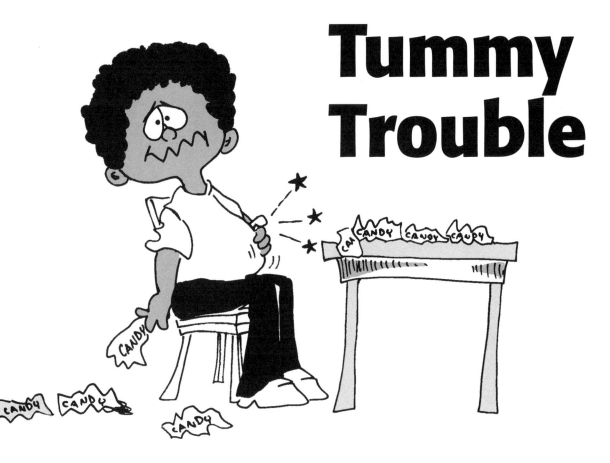

Tummy Trouble

Tummy aches can be caused by eating too much or spoiled food, stress, infection, or parasites.

Vomiting and diarrhea can cause children to lose body fluid and become dehydrated. Offer children sips of water or caffeine-free beverages to prevent dehydration. Gelatins and frozen ice pops are also good.

Call children's doctors if diarrhea or vomiting continues for more than one day (or sooner, for infants), or if children seem dehydrated.

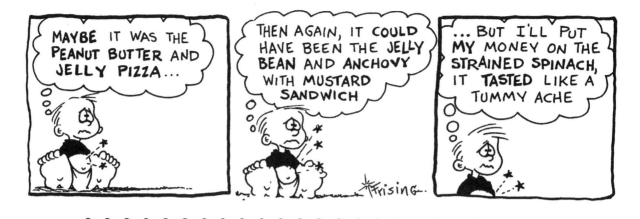

Tummy Trouble

Sometimes children have tummy aches, vomiting, or diarrhea. Tummy problems can be caused by eating too much or spoiled food, stress, infection, or parasites. Children may get stomachaches or diarrhea when taking antibiotics or other medicines.

Tummy problems that are not serious go away after a few hours. However, prolonged diarrhea and vomiting can cause dehydration. If children are vomiting or have diarrhea, give them small sips of clear liquids to replace the fluids lost. It is usually best to give water or clear fluids, such as caffeine-free flavored waters, gelatins, or frozen pops. Ask the children's doctors or a pharmacist about other liquids, such as sports drinks. If children cannot keep fluids down and have dry skin, sunken eyes, or are not urinating at least every six hours, call the doctor immediately.

When children feel like eating food again, offer crackers, toast, or plain soups, such as chicken noodle, for the first few meals. Milk, ice cream, fruit juice, or solid foods may cause stomach upsets.

If children continue to vomit or have diarrhea for more than twenty-four hours, or if you are worried, call their doctor. For infants, call a doctor after just a few hours. Infants can become seriously ill very quickly.

From *Hip on Health: Health Information for Caregivers and Families* by Charlotte M. Hendricks. Published by Redleaf Press. www.redleafpress.org.

Antibiotics

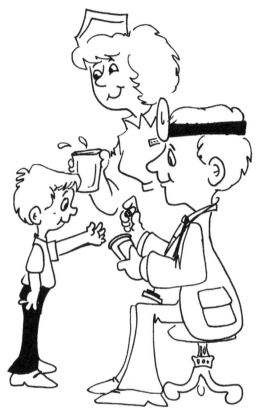

A doctor may prescribe antibiotics if a child has a bacterial infection. These powerful drugs kill the disease-causing bacteria.

Sometimes the child feels better after just a few doses of antibiotic. However, it takes the entire course of treatment to get rid of the infection. If the infection is not completely cured, the child may develop a more serious or drug-resistant infection.

It is important that the child take all of the prescribed antibiotic! This usually means taking medicine for 7 to 10 days.

From *Hip on Health: Health Information for Caregivers and Families* by Charlotte M. Hendricks. Published by Redleaf Press. www.redleafpress.org.

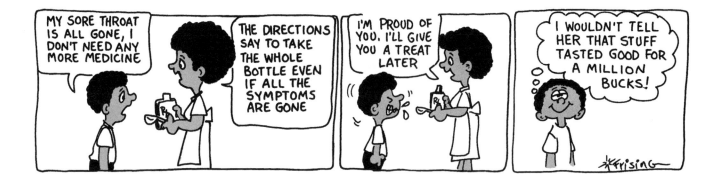

Antibiotics

If a child has a bacterial infection, the doctor may prescribe a specific type and amount of antibiotic. Antibiotics are powerful drugs that kill the disease-causing bacteria in the child's body. Antibiotics do not relieve symptoms, such as sore throat or fever. That is why a doctor may prescribe an antibiotic and another medicine such as acetaminophen or ibuprofen to help the child feel better.

Carefully give the correct amount of medicine. If the directions say to give one teaspoon, be sure you measure the medicine with a medicine dropper or the syringe that comes with the medicine. A regular spoon that you eat with may not measure the correct amount.

Often the child feels better after just a few doses of antibiotic. However, it takes the entire prescribed course of treatment to kill all the infection. It is important that the child take the entire amount of antibiotic! This usually means taking the medicine for seven to ten days.

If the bacterial infection is not completely eliminated, the child may develop a more serious infection. For example, if the child has strep throat, the sore throat may go away after just two or three days of antibiotics. However, if you stop the treatment then, bacteria remain. This can lead to a more serious infection, disease such as rheumatic fever, or an antibiotic-resistant infection.

From *Hip on Health: Health Information for Caregivers and Families* by Charlotte M. Hendricks. Published by Redleaf Press. www.redleafpress.org.

Calling the Doctor—Infants

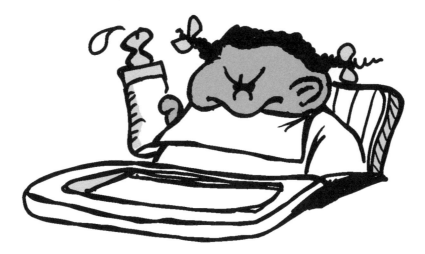

Infants can get very sick very quickly.

Trust your intuition. If you think something is wrong with an infant, call the child's doctor.

Do not wait! Even a few hours may make a difference in how well babies respond to treatment.

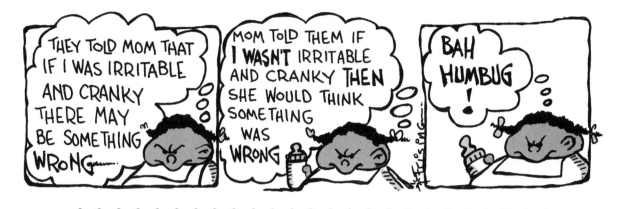

Calling the Doctor—Infants

Infants can get very sick very quickly. If you think something is wrong with an infant, call a doctor. Do not wait! Even a few hours may make a difference in how well infants respond to treatment. Here are some signs that medical care may be needed:

- ✓ Any fever in newborns up to three months. Fever above 100°F in older infants.

- ✓ Infants become "floppy," lose muscle tone, or seem to be very sick.

- ✓ Infants stop feeding normally.

- ✓ Infants cry for an unusually long time, are unusually cranky and irritable, or unusually sleepy.

- ✓ Breathing problems, including stuffy noses that prevent breathing while feeding.

- ✓ Vomiting in newborns (not spit-up). For older infants, forceful vomiting, vomiting that lasts for several hours, or vomit that is clear and fluid. Vomiting with fever or diarrhea.

- ✓ Diarrhea in newborns to three months old. For older infants, diarrhea with more than three episodes with severe abdominal cramps, or that appears watery.

- ✓ Dehydration, indicated by no wet diapers in six hours, dry, tacky mouth, or crying with few tears.

- ✓ Eyes that are pink, bloodshot, or have sticky discharge.

- ✓ Redness or tenderness around the navel area.

- ✓ White patches in the mouth.

Trust your intuition. If you are worried, call the child's doctor.

From *Hip on Health: Health Information for Caregivers and Families* by Charlotte M. Hendricks. Published by Redleaf Press. www.redleafpress.org.

Calling the Doctor— Young Children

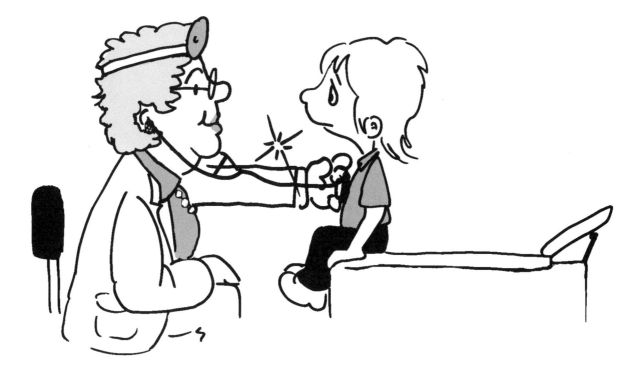

Trust your intuition. If you think a child is sick, call a doctor!

Call as soon as you notice symptoms, especially if the symptoms begin during the day when the doctor's office is open.

If you wait, you may end up in emergency care at night.

From *Hip on Health: Health Information for Caregivers and Families* by Charlotte M. Hendricks. Published by Redleaf Press. www.redleafpress.org.

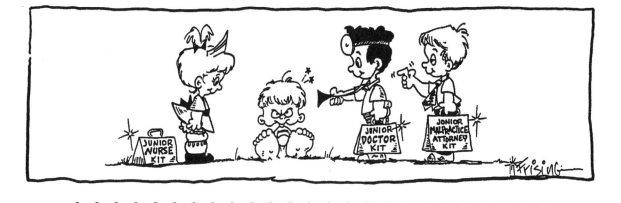

Calling the Doctor— Young Children

Trust your intuition. If you think a child is sick, call the doctor as soon as you notice symptoms. If you wait, you may end up in emergency care at night. Here are some signs that medical care may be needed:

✓ Temperature over 102°F or over 100°F when other symptoms are present.

✓ Shaking and chills.

✓ Extreme sleepiness or listlessness. Hysterical crying.

✓ Sudden weakness or paralysis. Seizures (convulsions).

✓ Loss of consciousness.

✓ Severe headache. Stiffness or pain in the neck.

✓ Earache or fluid from the ear.

✓ Sudden vision changes. Eyes that are red, swollen, and watery.

✓ Severe sore throat. Trouble swallowing or speaking.

✓ Breathing problems, rapid breathing, or severe cough.

✓ Vomiting for several hours or vomiting of blood.

✓ Intense or unusual abdominal pain or pain in the small of the back or either side.

✓ Diarrhea for several hours or diarrhea streaked with blood.

✓ Dehydration, indicated when children have not urinated in more than six hours, crying produces few tears, or mouth is dry.

✓ Pain, redness, or swelling of a joint. Wound that oozes pus or becomes hot, red, tender, or swollen.

From *Hip on Health: Health Information for Caregivers and Families* by Charlotte M. Hendricks. Published by Redleaf Press. www.redleafpress.org.

Going to the Hospital

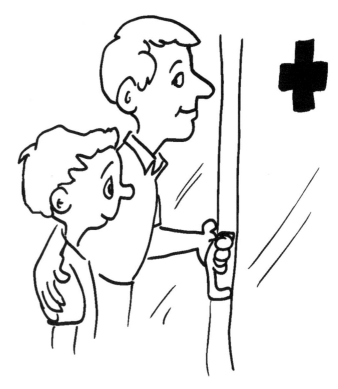

Going to the hospital can be frightening to children. Talk to them before you go. Explain what will be done in words that won't frighten them.

Take along a favorite toy, book, or crayons and paper so they can play while waiting.

Let them talk to the doctor or nurse and ask questions.

Stay with children and hold their hands and talk to them.

From *Hip on Health: Health Information for Caregivers and Families* by Charlotte M. Hendricks. Published by Redleaf Press. www.redleafpress.org.

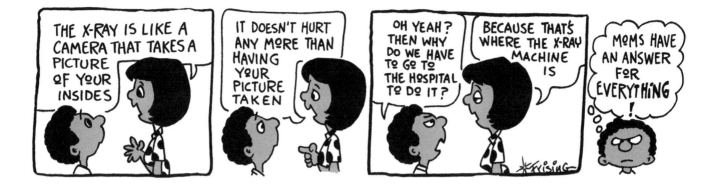

Going to the Hospital

Going to the hospital for tests or for an overnight stay can be frightening to children. Here are some ways to make the visit less frightening:

✓ Find out what kind of test will be done. Explain the test in words that will not frighten children. For example, if they are going to have X-rays, CT scans, or ultrasounds, explain that the machines are like a big special camera that can see through your skin and take pictures of the insides.

✓ Take a toy, book, or crayons and paper so children can play while waiting. A favorite doll or blanket helps calm fears.

✓ Explain how doctors, nurses, technicians, and other health helpers can find out how their bodies are working. These individuals can help keep people strong and well. Let children talk to the doctor or nurse and ask questions.

✓ Stay with children when possible. Holding their hands and talking to them will help. Most hospitals allow parents or guardians to stay in children's rooms.

Hospital visits can be frightening for adults too. Parents or caregivers cannot always stay with children during tests or after surgery. Find out when you can or cannot be with them. Ask for explanations about tests that will be done. Know what medicine children will be given, when they should get it, and why they are receiving it.

From *Hip on Health: Health Information for Caregivers and Families* by Charlotte M. Hendricks. Published by Redleaf Press. www.redleafpress.org.

Hand Washing

Many diseases are spread by direct contact. This means touching someone who is ill or touching an object that the ill person touched.

Germs can get on your hands and then enter your body when you touch your nose, mouth, or eyes.

Help prevent diseases by washing your hands. Wash hands before eating, after using the toilet, and after playtime.

Soap and running water are best for washing hands.

From *Hip on Health: Health Information for Caregivers and Families* by Charlotte M. Hendricks. Published by Redleaf Press. www.redleafpress.org.

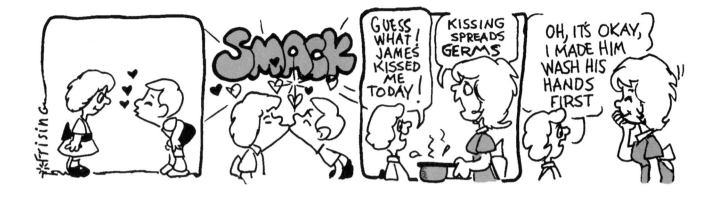

Hand Washing

Children share germs when they put their hands in their mouths, share toys, and get kissed. They cannot avoid all germs, but they can learn to help prevent the spread of germs that cause illness and infection.

The best way to prevent illness is to wash hands! Teach children to wash hands thoroughly with soap and water. Show them how to make soap bubbles and rub them all over hands, wrists, and between fingers. Check under fingernails for dirt too.

Rub hands with soapy lather for at least twenty seconds. Rinse hands under running water.

If you do not have soap and running water, premoistened wipes and waterless hand sanitizer help. These are not as good as soap and water.

Children watch you and learn from what you do. Wash your hands before eating or preparing food and after toileting.

When children are sick, wash your hands after helping them so you will not spread germs to other children or adults. Teach children to flush the toilet and wash their hands every time they use the toilet.

From *Hip on Health: Health Information for Caregivers and Families* by Charlotte M. Hendricks. Published by Redleaf Press. www.redleafpress.org.

Immunizations

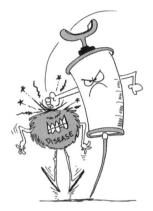

Immunizations are shots or medicines given by mouth that prevent diseases that are dangerous for children. Children should receive these immunizations:

- chicken pox
- rubella (German measles)
- rotavirus
- tetanus
- polio
- pertussis (whooping cough)
- measles
- hepatitis A and B
- mumps
- influenza (flu virus)
- diphtheria
- pneumococcal disease
- Hib (*Haemophilus influenza* type B)

For more information about immunizations, call your doctor or local health department, or visit www.cdc.gov/vaccines.

From *Hip on Health: Health Information for Caregivers and Families* by Charlotte M. Hendricks. Published by Redleaf Press. www.redleafpress.org.

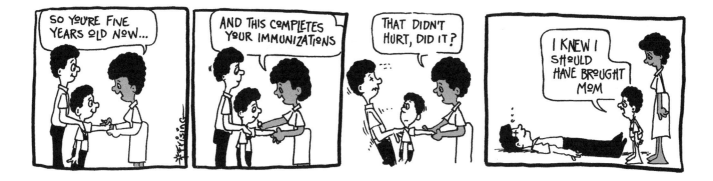

Immunizations

Immunizations can protect children against diseases that can make them very sick and be life threatening. Different immunizations are needed during the first five years of life. Recommended immunizations protect against these diseases:

✓ **Measles** causes fever, weakness, cough, and rash. It can cause breathing problems or convulsions.

✓ **Mumps** causes fever, headache, and earache. The glands on the side of the face may swell.

✓ **Rubella**, or German measles, causes fever, rash, and sore throat.

✓ **Diphtheria** affects the nose, throat, and skin. It can cause suffocation or paralysis and heart damage. Diphtheria can be fatal.

✓ **Tetanus**, or lockjaw, causes painful muscle contractions. It can be fatal.

✓ **Pertussis**, or whooping cough, causes continuous coughing that can last several weeks.

✓ **Chicken pox** causes fever and a rash and can affect internal organs.

✓ **Rotavirus** causes severe vomiting and diarrhea.

✓ **Polio** can cause paralysis, meningitis, and respiratory infections.

✓ **Hib (*Haemophilus influenzae*)** can cause ear infection, meningitis, pneumonia, and other complications.

✓ **Hepatitis A and B** affect the liver and can cause death.

✓ **Pneumococcal disease** is a respiratory infection that can cause meningitis or other complications.

✓ **Influenza** can cause serious complications. An annual flu vaccine is recommended.

From *Hip on Health: Health Information for Caregivers and Families* by Charlotte M. Hendricks. Published by Redleaf Press. www.redleafpress.org.

Know Your Medicine

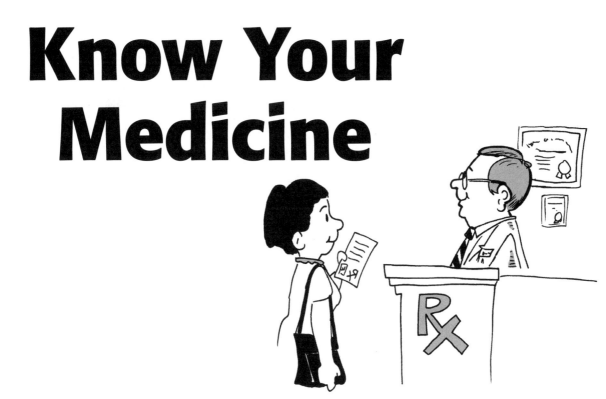

When children need medicine, be sure to ask the doctor or pharmacist these questions about it:

- What is the name of the medicine?

- How much should I give in each dose?

- Does the child need to take all the medicine? How many days?

- Will this medicine cause a stomachache, diarrhea, or other side effects?

If children react to the medicine or their symptoms become worse, call the doctor immediately.

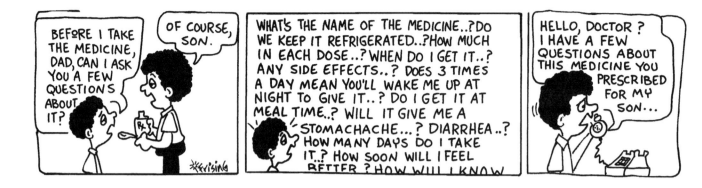

Know Your Medicine

When children are sick, their doctor may order a prescription medicine, such as an antibiotic, from a pharmacist. Over-the-counter (OTC) medicines, such as acetaminophen or first aid cream, can be purchased without a doctor's prescription.

It can be unsafe to take more than one kind of medicine. Do not give children medicine unless their doctor or pharmacist says it is okay. Tell the doctor about any other medicines children are taking.

Here are some questions to ask the doctor or pharmacist:

✓ What is the name of the medicine?

✓ Does it need to be kept in the refrigerator?

✓ How much should I give in each dose? When should I give it?

✓ Does "three times a day" mean I should wake the child at night for a dose?

✓ Should I give the medicine at mealtime? Are there any foods the child should not eat while taking this medicine?

✓ Will this medicine cause a stomachache, diarrhea, or other side effects?

✓ How will I know if the medicine is working?

✓ Should I bring the child back to see you after taking all the medicine?

✓ Does the child need to take all the medicine? For how many days?

If you think the medicine is not working or the children's symptoms become worse, call their doctor. If they have an adverse reaction to the medicine, call the doctor immediately.

From *Hip on Health: Health Information for Caregivers and Families* by Charlotte M. Hendricks. Published by Redleaf Press. www.redleafpress.org.

Medical Home

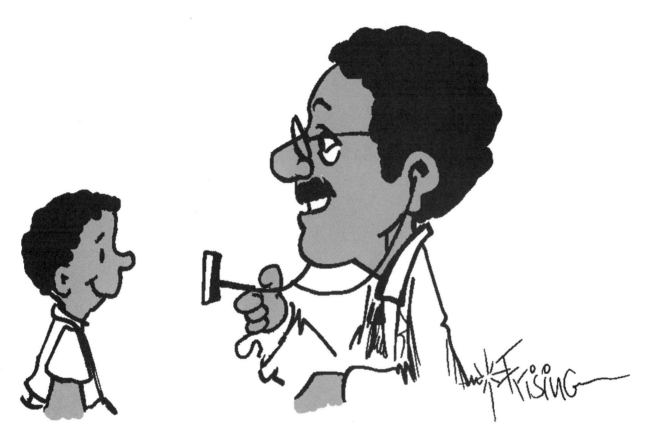

Children should have regular medical health care providers for consistent and regular health care. This is called a "Medical Home." The medical home may include doctors, nurse practitioners, and physicians' assistants. It may be a private doctor's office, a clinic, or a health department.

Regular and routine care allows health care providers to know each child better and provide the best health care.

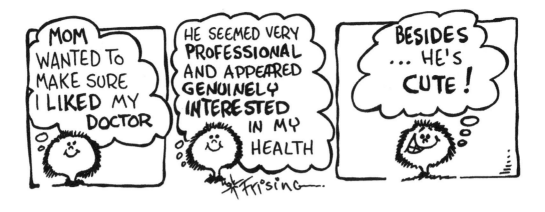

Medical Home

Children should have regular medical health care providers to provide consistent and regular health care. This is called a "Medical Home." The medical home may include doctors, nurse practitioners, and physicians' assistants. It may be a private doctor's office, a clinic, or a health department.

Regular health care promotes children's growth and development and helps prevent illness. The medical home staff keeps children's medical records and tells you when to schedule immunizations or well-child visits.

A medical home helps doctors and other health care professionals know each child better and provide the best care for each one.

Ask questions when choosing a medical home:

✓ What are the office hours? Does the clinic offer weekend and evening hours?

✓ Who will see children if their regular medical providers are not available?

✓ Which hospital will children go to if treatment is needed?

✓ How will you reach the medical provider after hours in an emergency?

✓ Is the waiting room set up so children with illnesses are separated from children who are there for well visits?

✓ Do you like the doctor and other staff? Does the child like the medical provider?

✓ Are you comfortable asking questions?

From *Hip on Health: Health Information for Caregivers and Families* by Charlotte M. Hendricks. Published by Redleaf Press. www.redleafpress.org.

Over-the-Counter Medicine

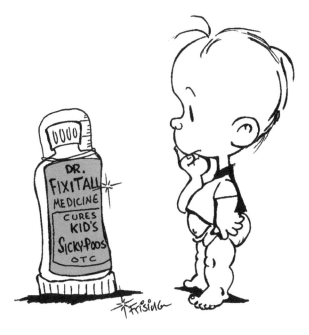

You can buy many medicines without a prescription. These are called over-the-counter (OTC) medicines. These products are safe for most people, when used correctly.

Talk to a doctor or pharmacist before giving medicine to children. Use the correct type for each child's age and weight.

Keep medicine in the original container. Read and follow the dosage instructions on the label.

From *Hip on Health: Health Information for Caregivers and Families* by Charlotte M. Hendricks. Published by Redleaf Press. www.redleafpress.org.

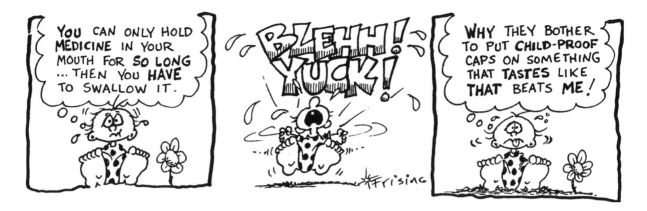

Over-the-Counter Medicine

If a child is ill or has symptoms, the child's doctor may tell you to give a specific medicine. Some medicines are available only by prescription. This means a doctor prescribes it, and you purchase it from a pharmacist.

Some medicine can be purchased without prescriptions. These are called over-the-counter (OTC) medicines. Many OTC medicines have the same ingredients as prescription drugs but may have a lower strength.

Many OTC products are sold under different names. Store brands may be less expensive than brand-name products. Look at the ingredients list. Both products should contain the same active ingredient and the same amount of that ingredient in each dose.

When used according to the label directions, OTC products are safe for most people. To use them effectively, follow these parameters:

✓ Talk to the doctor or pharmacist before giving any medicine to children.

✓ Some drugs' dosages are based on children's weight and age. A pharmacist can help you choose the correct type (such as pills or liquid) and dosage.

✓ Keep the medicine in its original labeled container.

✓ Read and follow the dosage instructions on the label. For liquids, use a medicine dropper or the syringe that is packaged with the medicine.

Watch for side effects or reactions to any medicine. Contact children's doctors if children have a reaction or seem to get worse.

From *Hip on Health: Health Information for Caregivers and Families* by Charlotte M. Hendricks. Published by Redleaf Press. www.redleafpress.org.

Pain and Fever Medicine

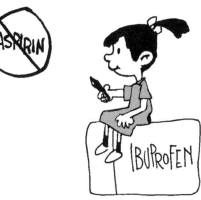

Two types of pain and fever medications can be recommended for young children.

- *Acetaminophen* is the active ingredient in products such as Tylenol.

- *Ibuprofen* is the ingredient in products such as Motrin, Advil, and Nuprin.

These medicines come in different forms and strengths. Ask a pharmacist to help you choose the correct type and dosage for children's age and weight. Keep medicine in the original package. Always read and follow the directions carefully.

Never give aspirin to children!

From *Hip on Health: Health Information for Caregivers and Families* by Charlotte M. Hendricks. Published by Redleaf Press. www.redleafpress.org.

155

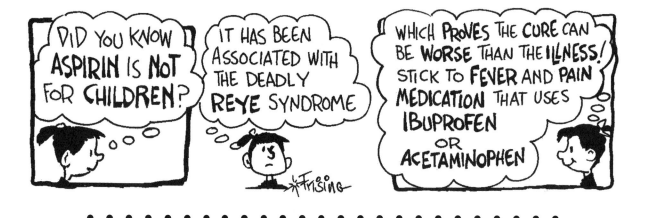

Pain and Fever Medicine

When children have low fevers but are playing, drinking fluids, and seem to feel well, then medicine probably is not needed for the fever. However, fever can make children ache, have headaches, or just feel bad. A doctor or pharmacist may recommend medicine to reduce children's fevers and help them feel better. Some medicines also help relieve pain.

There are two types of pain and fever medications recommended for young children. *Acetaminophen* is the active ingredient in products such as Tylenol. *Ibuprofen* is the ingredient in products such as Motrin. Generics and store brands of these medicines are just as good and may be less expensive.

Acetaminophen and ibuprofen have few side effects and are safe when used as directed. Be sure you give the correct type and dosage for children's age and weight!

These medicines may come in drops for infants, liquid ("elixir") and chewable tablets for toddlers, and junior-strength chewable tablets for older children. Use the right type for the child's age and weight!

Keep medicine in the original package. Always read and follow the directions carefully.

Naproxen, the ingredient in products such as Aleve, can be recommended for older children and teenagers.

Never give aspirin to children or teenagers. Aspirin has been associated with the development of Reye syndrome, a rare but life-threatening condition.

From *Hip on Health: Health Information for Caregivers and Families* by Charlotte M. Hendricks. Published by Redleaf Press. www.redleafpress.org.

Stop Germs

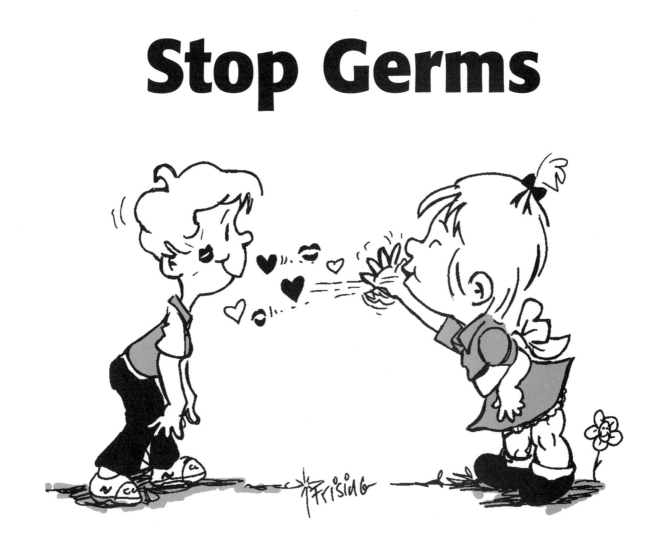

Children pick up germs everywhere. The most important way to avoid germs and prevent disease is to wash hands.

Teach children to wash their hands thoroughly with soap and water. It is especially important to wash hands after using the toilet and before preparing food and eating.

Germs can be spread by kissing. Teach children how to "blow a kiss" and avoid those germs.

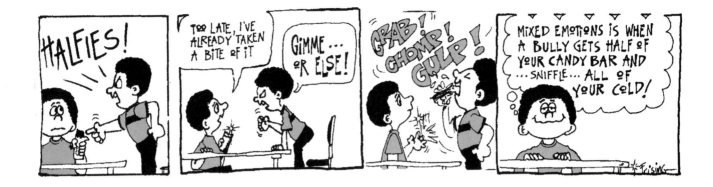

Stop Germs

Children pick up germs everywhere. Everything they touch, such as doorknobs and grocery cart handles, has germs. They get germs from friends, brothers and sisters, and you! Even children who stay at home are exposed to germs from family members.

Not all germs are bad. But some cause illness, such as colds, runny noses, diarrhea, and tummy problems. Some germs cause more serious problems.

The best way to prevent disease is to wash hands! Teach children to wash their hands often and thoroughly with soap and running water. It is especially important for them to wash hands after using the toilet and before preparing food and eating.

Children share germs when they share food or drinks. Teach them how to share food the healthy way. For example, they can pour a drink into separate glasses before tasting it.

Many adults and children love to kiss infants. But infants can get sick from germs. For example, the herpes virus that causes cold sores in adults can cause serious medical problems in infants.

Avoid kissing infants on the mouth or hands (since hands usually go straight into their mouths). Even better—encourage children to "blow a kiss" and avoid those germs completely!

From *Hip on Health: Health Information for Caregivers and Families* by Charlotte M. Hendricks. Published by Redleaf Press. www.redleafpress.org.

Throw Away Old Medicine

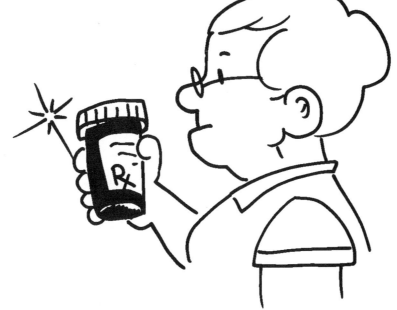

Medicines can lose their strength or change chemically when they get too old. Throw away prescription medicines one year after the purchase date. Liquid antibiotics are good for about two weeks only.

When using over-the-counter (nonprescription) medicines, look for the expiration date on the label. Throw medicines away after the expiration date. If you do not see an expiration date or do not know how old medicine is, throw it away.

From *Hip on Health: Health Information for Caregivers and Families* by Charlotte M. Hendricks. Published by Redleaf Press. www.redleafpress.org.

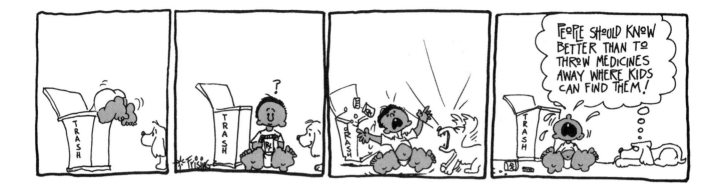

Throw Away Old Medicine

Medicines should be stored out of children's sight and out of reach. Keep them in their original bottles with child-resistant caps. Medicines prescribed for one person should never be given to anyone else.

It is important to store medicines properly. Keep them in a cool, dry, and dark place. A locked cabinet or box high in a closet works well. Some liquid medicines can be stored in the refrigerator. Do not keep medicines out in bathrooms or kitchens. Heat, steam, and sunlight can ruin them.

Some medicines lose their strength when they get too old. Other medicines may change and become dangerous to use. Throw away prescription medicines one year after the purchase date. Liquid antibiotics are good for about two weeks only.

When using over-the-counter (nonprescription) medicines, look for the expiration date on the label. Throw medicines away after the expiration date. If you do not see an expiration date or do not know how old medicine is, throw it away.

Do not throw medicines in the trash where children might find them. Ask your pharmacist how to dispose of medicine safely.

From *Hip on Health: Health Information for Caregivers and Families* by Charlotte M. Hendricks. Published by Redleaf Press. www.redleafpress.org.

Visiting the Doctor

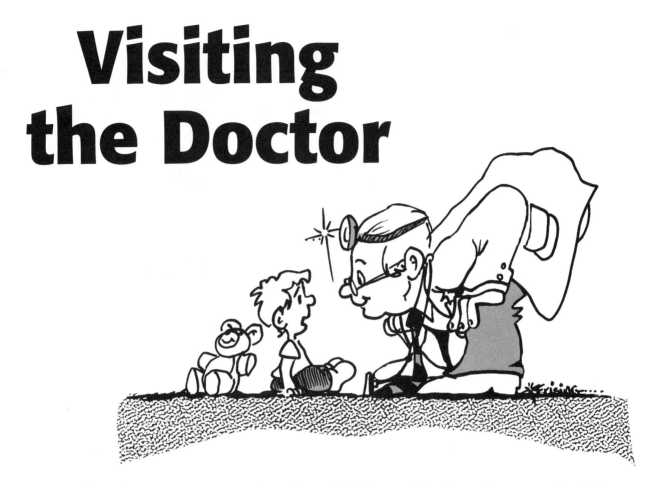

Visits to the doctor are easier for children if they know what to expect. Talk to them about why they are going. People go to a doctor when they are sick. They also go when they are well for checkups.

Discuss what the doctor or nurse will do. Help them understand that doctors and nurses are health helpers.

If children are scared of the doctor or nurse, they may not behave well. Never threaten them with going to the doctor. Do not scare them with talk about shots or needles.

From *Hip on Health: Health Information for Caregivers and Families* by Charlotte M. Hendricks. Published by Redleaf Press. www.redleafpress.org.

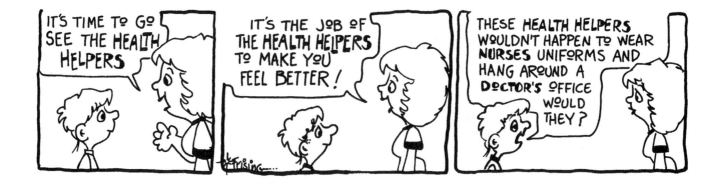

Visiting the Doctor

Children visit doctors for checkups and when they are sick. Visits are easier when children know what to expect. Talk to them before going. Help them understand that doctors and nurses are health helpers.

Children who are scared of doctors or nurses may not behave well. Try to understand their fears and talk about them. Never threaten children with going to the doctor. Do not scare them with talk about shots or needles.

Make a list of sick children's symptoms, such as fever, stomachache, sore throat, sneezing, diarrhea, and behavior changes. Tell the doctor how long they have had these symptoms.

You can help children feel better if you know what to expect. Ask questions such as these:

✓ What is the name of the illness? How long will it last?

✓ Will medicine help the child get well faster?

✓ What other symptoms should I expect, and how long will they last? Are there any serious symptoms I should watch for?

✓ Will the child have a fever? What temperature (fever) is too high?

✓ What can I do to make the child feel better?

✓ Is the illness contagious? Can the child go back to child care or school with this illness?

✓ What can I do to prevent this illness again?

From *Hip on Health: Health Information for Caregivers and Families* by Charlotte M. Hendricks. Published by Redleaf Press. www.redleafpress.org.

Well-Child Checkups

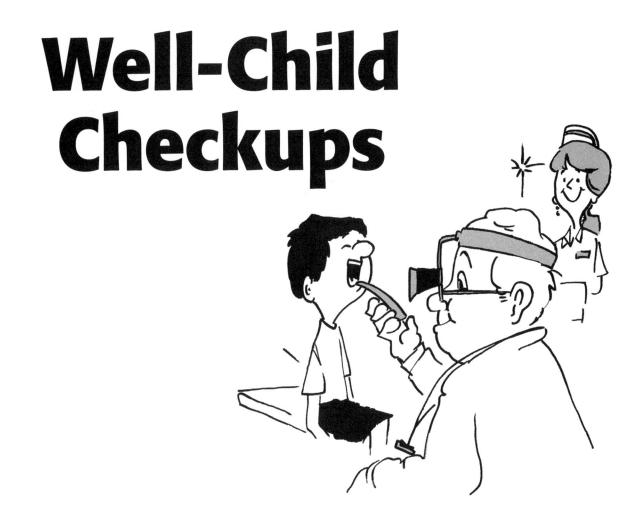

Even when children are healthy, well-child visits for preventive care are important to keep them healthy.

Each visit includes a complete head-to-toe physical examination. The doctor checks and records children's growth, development, and other important information. Hearing, vision, and other screening tests occur during some visits.

Some visits include immunizations to protect children against diseases such as measles, mumps, and chicken pox.

From *Hip on Health: Health Information for Caregivers and Families* by Charlotte M. Hendricks. Published by Redleaf Press. www.redleafpress.org.

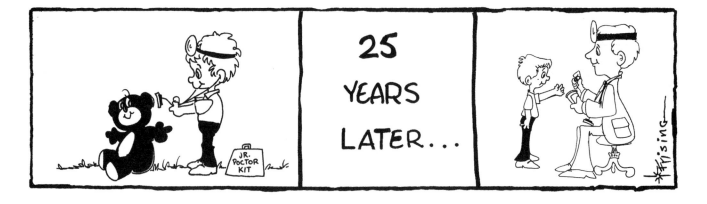

Well-Child Checkups

Childhood is a time of rapid growth and change, and even when children are healthy, well-child visits to a doctor for preventive care are important to check on their development.

The American Academy of Pediatrics recommends that parents, especially first-time parents, visit with a health care provider *before* their infant is born. The next visit probably occurs when infants are a few days old. After that, regular well-child visits are usually recommended at the following ages:

1 month	2 months	4 months
6 months	9 months	1 year
15 months	18 months	2 years
2½ years	3 years	4 years

and once every year after that.

Each visit includes a complete head-to-toe physical examination. The doctor checks and records children's growth, development, and other important information. Hearing, vision, and other screening tests occur during some visits.

Immunizations are given when they are due to ensure that children are protected against diseases such as measles, mumps, and chicken pox.

Well-child visits are key times for communication. Parents or guardians are usually given information about children's normal development, nutrition, sleep, safety, and diseases that are going around. Health care providers may also discuss other important topics, such as family relationships, child care and school, and access to community services.

Before going for the well-child visits, write down any questions and concerns they have. In addition to these, visits to health care providers should be scheduled anytime children seem ill or adults are worried about children's health or development.

From *Hip on Health: Health Information for Caregivers and Families* by Charlotte M. Hendricks. Published by Redleaf Press. www.redleafpress.org.

Back to Sleep

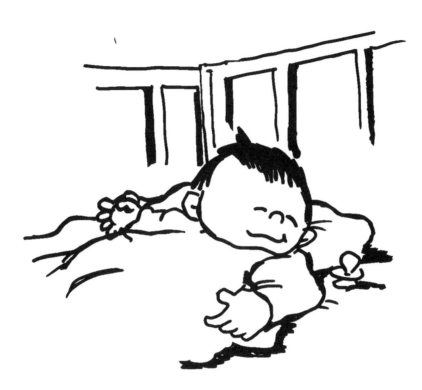

Healthy infants should be placed on their backs to sleep. This position keeps their noses and mouths uncovered. Sleeping on their stomachs can push infants' faces into bedding, blocking their breathing passages.

Be sure infants are placed on their backs to sleep, at home and in child care.

From *Hip on Health: Health Information for Caregivers and Families* by Charlotte M. Hendricks. Published by Redleaf Press. www.redleafpress.org.

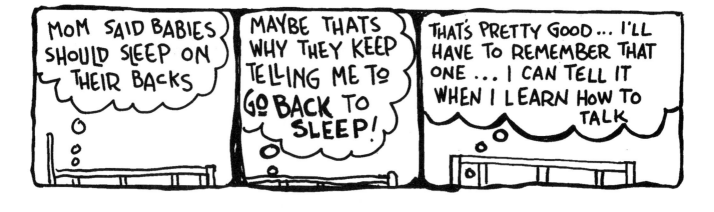

Back to Sleep

Healthy infants should be placed on their backs to sleep. Sleeping on their stomachs may push infants' faces into the bedding, blocking their breathing passages. Sleeping on their backs keeps their noses and mouths uncovered. This is important at home and in child care.

Healthy infants are not in danger of spitting up or choking while sleeping on their backs. In fact, the incidence of Sudden Infant Death Syndrome (SIDS) has decreased by over 50 percent since the Back-to-Sleep campaign (now called "Safe Sleep") began in 1994.

As infants grow older, they may turn over and sleep on their tummies sometimes. This is okay. It is still important that they be placed on their backs when put in cribs.

Infants with certain medical conditions or malformations may need to be placed on their sides or stomachs. Their doctor will tell you if infants should sleep in a different position.

Infants need lots of tummy time while they are awake. Tummy time helps promote muscle and motor development. Infants who stay on their back all the time (even when awake) can develop flat areas on the backs of their heads. Tummy time helps prevent this.

From *Hip on Health: Health Information for Caregivers and Families* by Charlotte M. Hendricks. Published by Redleaf Press. www.redleafpress.org.

Bottle Sanitation

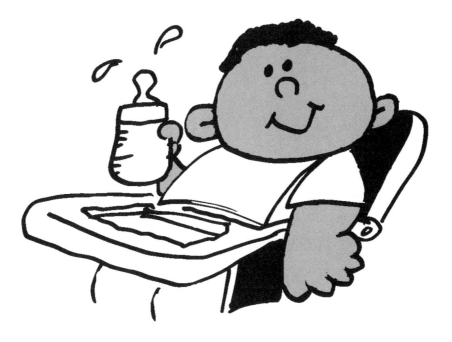

One of the most enjoyable moments is holding and cuddling infants during bottle feeding. Make sure there are no harmful bacteria or germs in the bottle. Follow these guidelines:

- Use a fresh bottle for each feeding. Complete feedings within one hour.

- Do not leave a bottle out of refrigeration for more than one hour.

- Clean bottles and nipples carefully before each use.

From *Hip on Health: Health Information for Caregivers and Families* by Charlotte M. Hendricks. Published by Redleaf Press. www.redleafpress.org.

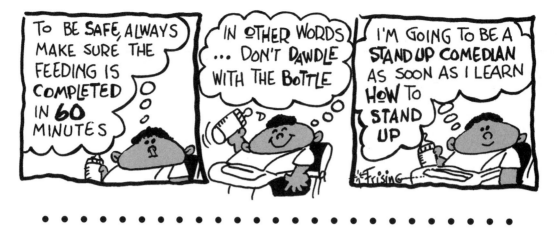

Bottle Sanitation

One of the most enjoyable moments is holding and cuddling infants during bottle feeding. For infants, bottles represent love, warmth, a full tummy, and a satisfying burp! Make sure bottles provide nourishment and not harmful germs.

Use a fresh bottle for each feeding. Bottles should be prepared with just enough breast milk or formula for a single feeding. Once infants' mouths touch the bottle, microorganisms from their mouths mix with the milk and can multiply and become harmful. Refrigeration or reheating will not prevent contamination.

Infants' feeding should be completed within one hour. After sixty minutes, harmful bacteria can have replicated in large numbers with the liquid at room temperature. Throw away unfinished formula or breast milk. Do not leave bottles out of refrigeration (such as in a diaper bag) for more than one hour.

Carefully clean bottles and nipples before each use. They can be cleaned in an automatic dishwasher or with hot soapy water. Rinse and air-dry. Be sure the hole in the nipple is cleaned thoroughly.

If infants have infections such as thrush, sterilize bottles, nipples, and pacifiers by placing in boiling water for five minutes. Remember—keep children out of the kitchen while you are sterilizing bottles!

From *Hip on Health: Health Information for Caregivers and Families* by Charlotte M. Hendricks. Published by Redleaf Press. www.redleafpress.org.

Bottle Warming

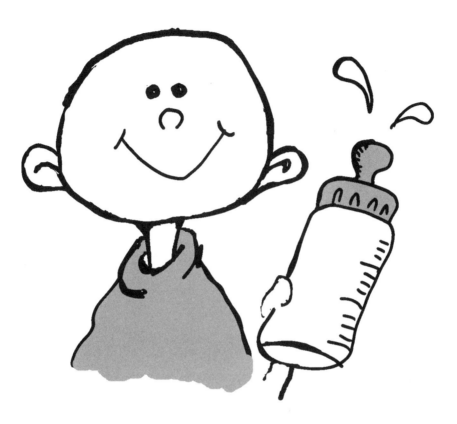

Infants' mouths and skin are very sensitive. They can become seriously burned when bottles are overheated.

Breast milk or formula can be served cold or at room temperature. Warming is not necessary.

If bottles are warmed, shake them after warming. Test the temperature on the back of your hand.

From *Hip on Health: Health Information for Caregivers and Families* by Charlotte M. Hendricks. Published by Redleaf Press. www.redleafpress.org.

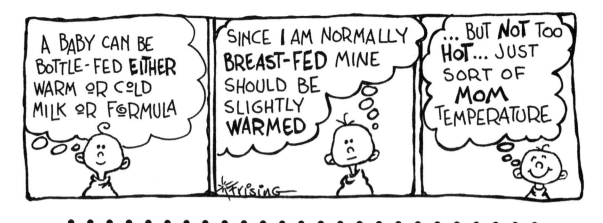

Bottle Warming

Infants' mouths and skin are very sensitive. They can become seriously burned when bottles are overheated. You must be very careful when heating bottles.

Bottles do not need to be warmed. Breast milk or formula can be served cold or at room temperature. However, if infants are normally breast fed, they are accustomed to milk that is body temperature. Therefore, they may be more willing to accept bottles that are warmed slightly.

To warm a bottle, place it in pan of warm water (no more than 120°F) for five minutes or less. Frozen breast milk should be thawed in a refrigerator about twelve hours before using.

Always shake the bottle after warming to prevent hot spots. Check the temperature by shaking a few drops onto the back of your hand. It should feel cool or slightly warm. If it feels warm to you, then it is probably too hot for infants.

Do not microwave bottles. There are many reported cases of serious burns to infants because of microwaved bottles.

Do not leave bottles out of refrigeration for more than one hour. After sixty minutes, harmful bacteria can grow.

From *Hip on Health: Health Information for Caregivers and Families* by Charlotte M. Hendricks. Published by Redleaf Press. www.redleafpress.org.

Crib Safety

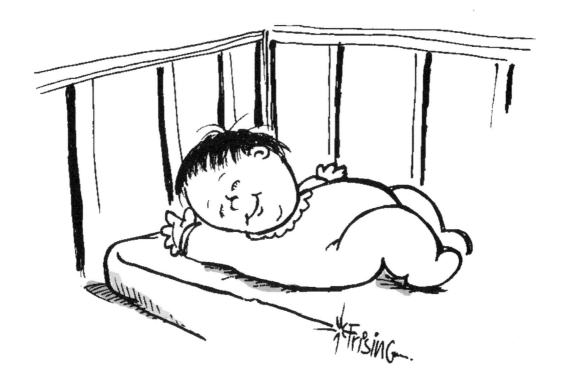

All infants should have their own beds. When they sleep in their own cribs, they get more sleep—and so do their parents! Infants should not sleep with adults or other children. Larger persons could roll over and suffocate or injure them.

Never put infants on beanbags, waterbeds, feather beds, or soft comforters or cushions. These can suffocate infants whose noses become blocked.

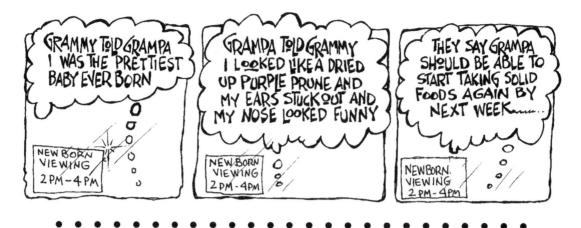

Crib Safety

All infants should have their own beds. When they sleep in their own cribs, they get more sleep—and so do the parents! Infants should not sleep with adults or older children. Larger persons could roll over and injure or suffocate infants.

Make sure infants' cribs are safe. Follow these guidelines:

✓ Check for openings that could trap infants' heads. There should be no more than 2³/8 inches between crib railings.

✓ Cribs should have solid headboards and footboards; cut-out openings could trap infants' heads.

✓ Corner posts must not protrude more than ¹/16 inch above the headboard or footboard.

✓ Check hardware regularly; be sure it is secure and tightened. Be sure there are no screws or bolts sticking out or any protrusion that could catch clothing.

✓ Watch for peeling paint, splinters, or rough edges.

Help avoid suffocation. Use properly fitted crib sheets that do not come loose. Dress infants in footed pajamas and only use small lightweight blankets, if necessary. Avoid heavy blankets or comforters. Do not place pillows or stuffed toys in the crib.

Never put infants on beanbags, pillows, waterbeds, feather beds, or soft comforters or cushions. These can suffocate infants if their noses become blocked.

From *Hip on Health: Health Information for Caregivers and Families* by Charlotte M. Hendricks. Published by Redleaf Press. www.redleafpress.org.

Crying

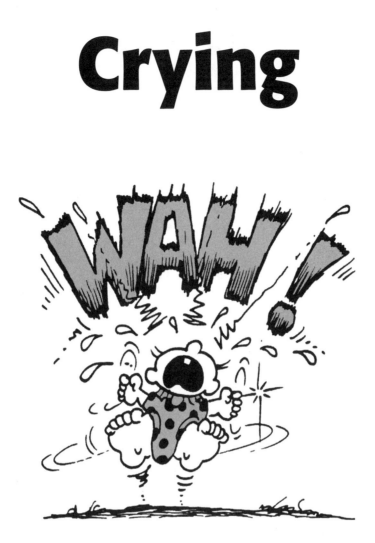

Infants cry when something is wrong. They may cry if they are hungry, wet, hot or cold, need to burp, tired, ill, or just lonely.

Always check on infants when they cry. Do not let them cry for more than 10 minutes without trying to comfort them. This nurturing from you makes them feel more secure and helps promote healthy brain development.

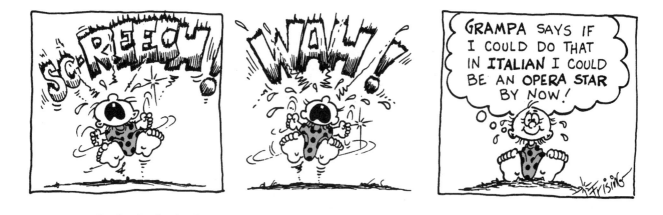

Crying

Infants communicate by crying: it means something is wrong. They may cry if they are hungry, wet, hot or cold, need to burp, tired, ill, or just lonely. Try to find out why they are crying and take care of their needs.

If they appear to be okay but are still crying, try to comfort them. Here are some suggestions:

✓ Give them a pacifier.

✓ Try to burp them.

✓ Try holding them in different positions.

✓ Gently rub their tummy with your warm hand.

✓ Rock or walk with them, providing gentle movement.

✓ Provide quiet music or white noise.

✓ Talk, sing, or hum to them.

Always check on crying infants. This nurturing from you makes them feel more secure and helps promote healthy brain development. Do not let them cry for more than ten minutes without trying to comfort them. Do not let them cry continuously.

If they are crying excessively and cannot be comforted, call their doctor. Infants can become very sick very quickly, and continual crying may be the first sign of illness.

From *Hip on Health: Health Information for Caregivers and Families* by Charlotte M. Hendricks. Published by Redleaf Press. www.redleafpress.org.

Diaper Rash

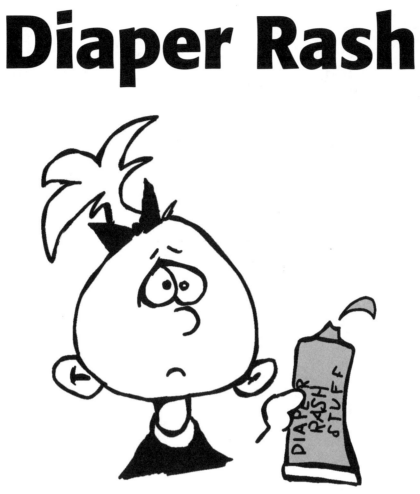

Help prevent diaper rash by following these guidelines:

- Change infants' diapers as soon as they are wet or soiled.

- Clean infants' bottoms during each diaper change.

- When possible, allow children to be diaper free.

- If you use cloth diapers, wash them in dye-free and fragrance-free detergent.

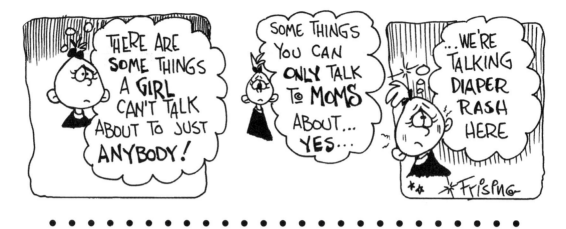

Diaper Rash

Most infants have diaper rash at some time. Diaper rash is usually caused by not changing soiled diapers quickly or often enough. It also can be caused by diarrhea. Soap and fabric softener in cloth diapers and chemicals that increase absorbency in disposable diapers may lead to skin irritation. Here are ways to treat and prevent diaper rash:

✓ Change infants' diapers as soon as they are wet or soiled.

✓ Clean infants' bottoms with each diaper change. Wipe from front to back, especially on girls. Clean with water and mild soap (if needed). Premoistened wipes can cause further irritation.

✓ Allow the skin to dry completely after cleaning.

✓ When possible, allow children to be diaper-free.

✓ Wash cloth diapers in dye-free and fragrance-free detergent.

✓ If you use disposable diapers and infants continue to have diaper rashes, try changing brands.

✓ Diaper creams usually are not needed. Ask children's doctors or pharmacists for a recommendation.

Baby powder is not recommended because it can be inhaled and cause respiratory distress. Keep powder out of infants' reach!

Diaper rash usually heals in three to four days. Contact children's doctors if rashes last more than three days, are worse in the creases at the top of the thighs, or are spreading and getting worse.

From *Hip on Health: Health Information for Caregivers and Families* by Charlotte M. Hendricks. Published by Redleaf Press. www.redleafpress.org.

Lifting Infants

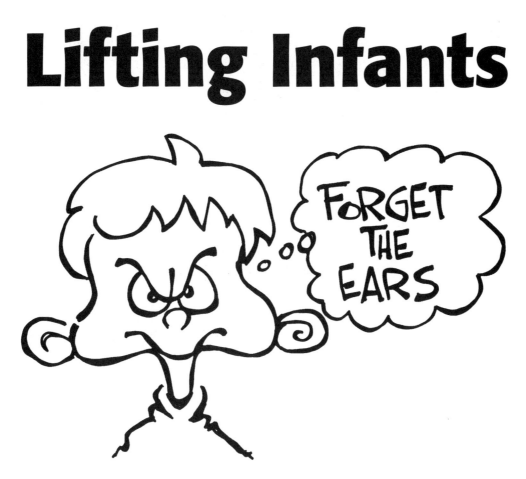

Infants and young children can be seriously injured if picked up incorrectly.

Firmly support their heads and necks when holding, lifting, or carrying young infants. Hold them securely and close to your body.

Do not toss infants into the air. Do not allow young children to hold or carry infants without adult assistance.

When lifting infants or young children, lift them securely under both arms.

From *Hip on Health: Health Information for Caregivers and Families* by Charlotte M. Hendricks. Published by Redleaf Press. www.redleafpress.org.

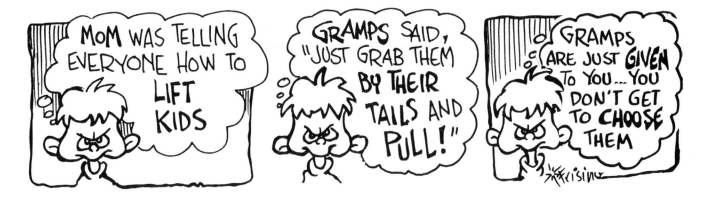

Lifting Infants

Infants and young children can be injured if they are picked up incorrectly. Jarring or jerky movements can cause injury to their necks, joints, muscles, and ligaments. Remember these tips when lifting infants and young children:

✓ Newborn infants have no control over head movements. Firmly support their heads and necks when holding, lifting, or carrying them.

✓ Hold infants securely and close to your body.

✓ Do not toss infants into the air!

✓ Children should not hold or carry infants without adult assistance.

✓ When lifting infants and young children, lift them securely under both arms. This supports and distributes their full body weight while they are lifted.

Lifting children by one arm or even by both arms can cause injury. Nursemaid's elbow is a common injury in toddlers and young children. In this injury, the radius (one of the bones in the forearm) pops out of place. This can occur if children's arms are pulled and twisted at the wrong angle, such as when children are improperly lifted by one arm. It can also occur children are swung by the arms or when children pull and twist to get away from your grasp.

From *Hip on Health: Health Information for Caregivers and Families* by Charlotte M. Hendricks. Published by Redleaf Press. www.redleafpress.org.

Shaken Baby Syndrome

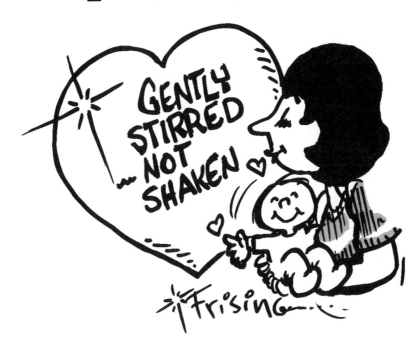

Never shake infants or children for any reason!

When an infant or child is shaken, the violent movement to the head bumps the brain against the skull. This can tear blood vessels and nerves in the brain, causing the brain to swell.

Shaking young children can cause intellectual disability, speech and learning disabilities, behavioral problems, cerebral palsy, paralysis, seizures, hearing loss, blindness, even death.

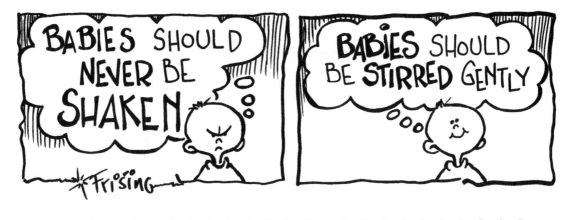

Shaken Baby Syndrome

Never shake infants or children for any reason. Shaken Baby Syndrome (SBS) is a leading cause of death from child abuse in the United States.

Vigorous shaking of infants or young children can result in injuries to arms, legs, chest, or shoulders. In some cases, shaking is followed by children's heads hitting a bed, chair, wall, floor, or other hard surface. The resulting injuries can be as severe as if children had fallen from a third story window.

Why is shaking young children so dangerous? Their muscles provide little or no support for their heads. When someone shakes them, the violent movement bumps their brains against their skulls. This can tear blood vessels and nerves in the brain, causing it to swell.

Shaking can also cause neck injury, intellectual disability, speech and learning disabilities, behavioral problems, cerebral palsy, paralysis, seizures, hearing loss, blindness, permanent vegetative state, and death.

Never toss infants or young children into the air! The jarring motion can lead to head and neck injuries. They also can be injured by hitting a hard surface, such as the ceiling, ceiling fan, wall, or floor.

From *Hip on Health: Health Information for Caregivers and Families* by Charlotte M. Hendricks. Published by Redleaf Press. www.redleafpress.org.

Solid Foods

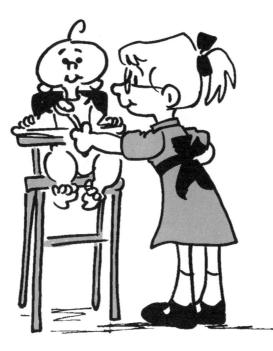

Infants and toddlers need to eat about every three hours.

Offer small portions of nutritious foods; add more if they're interested. If they turn their heads away or push food away, let them stop eating.

Young children can easily choke on foods that are round, slippery, dry, tough, sticky, or hard. Foods with nonedible parts, such as fish with bones and fruits with pits, are also dangerous.

From *Hip on Health: Health Information for Caregivers and Families* by Charlotte M. Hendricks. Published by Redleaf Press. www.redleafpress.org.

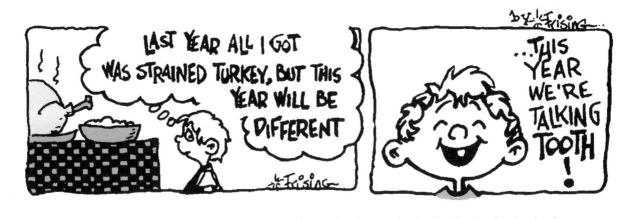

Solid Foods

For the first year of life, infants should get most of their nutrition from breast milk or formula. Their doctors will recommend when to start giving solid food, usually at about four months. Doctors often recommend cereals first, followed by other single-ingredient baby foods.

Try each new food for several days before introducing another one. As you introduce new foods, watch for signs of food allergy or intolerance. Talk to children's doctors if tummy aches, diarrhea, rashes, sneezes, or other physical symptoms occur after children eat certain foods.

At the toddler stage, children's growth slows down, but toddlers still need to eat about every three hours. Most active toddlers need three small meals and two snacks each day.

Toddlers have unpredictable eating habits. They may eat well one day and then be picky eaters for a day or two. Offer them small portions of nutritious foods; add more if they are interested. If children turn their heads away or push food away, let them stop eating. Do not force them to eat.

Young children can easily choke on foods that are round, slippery, dry, tough, sticky, or hard. Hot dogs and grapes can easily cause choking. Foods with nonedible parts, such as fish with bones or fruits with pits, also are dangerous. Cut or finely chop such foods, or simply wait to introduce some foods until children are older.

From *Hip on Health: Health Information for Caregivers and Families* by Charlotte M. Hendricks. Published by Redleaf Press. www.redleafpress.org.

Breakfast

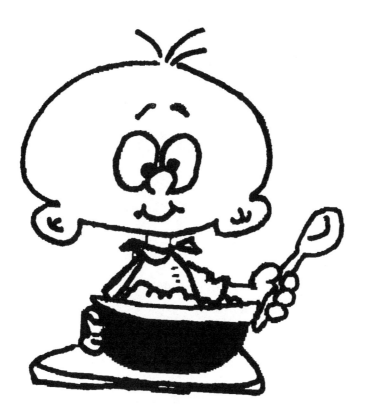

Eating a nutritious breakfast every day promotes healthy growth and development and helps children do their best all morning.

Choose nutritious foods that children enjoy and serve these for breakfast. These might be oatmeal, spaghetti, a peanut butter and jelly sandwich, or a hamburger!

Make lower-sugar cereal by mixing sweetened and unsweetened cereals.

From *Hip on Health: Health Information for Caregivers and Families* by Charlotte M. Hendricks. Published by Redleaf Press. www.redleafpress.org.

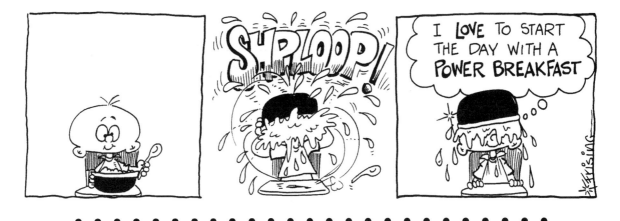

Breakfast

Breakfast is the most important meal of the day for children. Their tummies are empty after a night's rest, and they need nutritious food to recharge themselves. Eating a nutritious breakfast every day promotes healthy growth and development and helps children do their best all morning.

Serve nutritious foods that children enjoy for breakfast. These may be oatmeal, eggs, cereal, spaghetti, a peanut butter and jelly sandwich, or a hamburger! Try making cheese toast: put a slice of a favorite cheese on whole wheat bread and toast it in the oven. Toasted cheese on crackers is good too!

Hot cereals are good. However, some instant hot cereals are high in sugar. Consider buying plain cereals and adding your own flavors. Put fresh or canned fruit pieces or applesauce in oatmeal. Add cheese to grits. Mix one packet of flavored oatmeal with one packet of plain.

If children prefer cold cereal, buy lower-sugar or unsweetened varieties and sweeten them with fruit. Make lower-sugar cereal by mixing sweetened and unsweetened cereals.

From *Hip on Health: Health Information for Caregivers and Families* by Charlotte M. Hendricks. Published by Redleaf Press. www.redleafpress.org.

Calcium

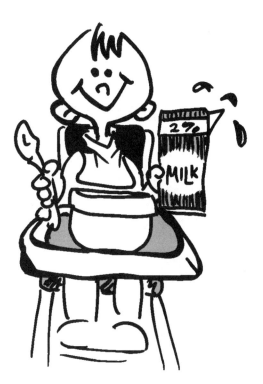

Children need calcium to develop strong bones and teeth. Calcium also helps their hearts, muscles, nerves, and blood flow.

Many foods contain calcium: milk and other dairy products, such as yogurt, pudding, and cheese, calcium-fortified orange juice, and some breakfast cereals and breads (fortified with calcium).

From *Hip on Health: Health Information for Caregivers and Families* by Charlotte M. Hendricks. Published by Redleaf Press. www.redleafpress.org.

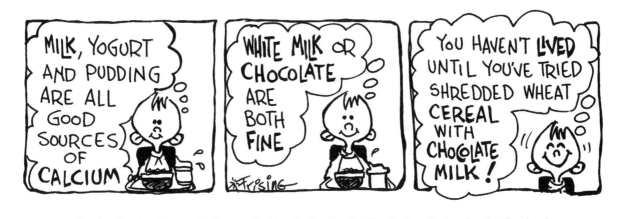

Calcium

Children need calcium to develop strong bones and teeth. Calcium also helps their hearts, muscles, and nerves.

Many children do not get enough calcium in their diets. Often, children avoid milk and choose sodas (soft drinks) or high-sugar juice boxes and miss out on calcium.

After one year of age, toddlers usually switch from breast milk or formula to cow's milk. Toddlers need fat in their diets for development, so they should drink whole milk until they are two years old. Then they can usually switch to low-fat or nonfat milk.

Dairy products such as yogurt, pudding, and cheese contain calcium, as do calcium-fortified orange juice (contains as much calcium as milk), some breakfast cereals and breads, tofu and certain types of beans (excellent sources of calcium), and dark green leafy vegetables.

Notice what children eat to see if they are getting enough calcium every day.

From *Hip on Health: Health Information for Caregivers and Families* by Charlotte M. Hendricks. Published by Redleaf Press. www.redleafpress.org.

Foodborne Illness

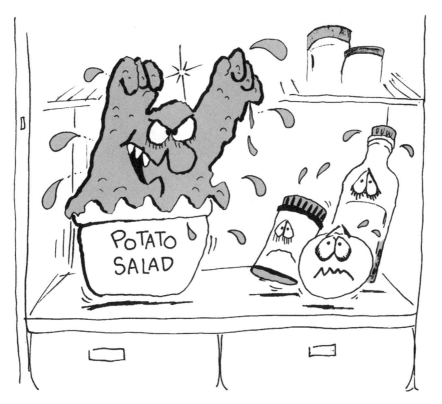

Prevent germs from growing in food.

Keep hot foods hot and cold foods cold.

Do not leave food at room temperature for more than two hours.

Cook foods until they are completely done. Do not eat pink meat or raw eggs.

Carefully clean countertops, cutting boards, knives, and other utensils before and after preparing foods.

From *Hip on Health: Health Information for Caregivers and Families* by Charlotte M. Hendricks. Published by Redleaf Press. www.redleafpress.org.

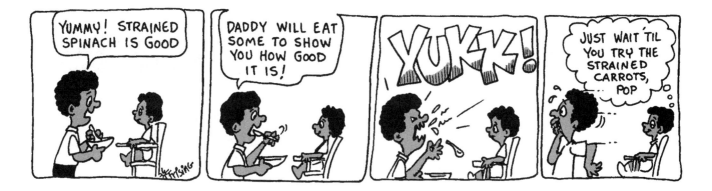

Foodborne Illness

Spoiled food can cause anything from a bad stomachache to life-threatening illness. Some disease-causing bacteria can grow in food. When eaten, some microorganisms can cause infections, nausea, fever, vomiting, and diarrhea.

Here are ways to keep food safe:

✓ Keep refrigerator temperatures below 40°F. Put meats, poultry, milk, and other cold foods in the refrigerator as soon as you get home from the store.

✓ Never leave milk and dairy foods, meat, eggs, or cooked foods at room temperature for more than two hours.

✓ Thaw frozen meats or poultry in the refrigerator.

✓ Cook poultry, beef, and pork until no pink remains.

✓ Cook eggs completely. Do not eat raw eggs or foods with raw eggs.

✓ When storing leftovers, cool hot food quickly. Put hot food in small containers and put it in the refrigerator or freezer so it will cool fast.

✓ Carefully wash countertops, cutting boards, knives, and other utensils after handling raw meat or poultry. Wash wooden cutting boards with hot soapy water and a little bleach.

From *Hip on Health: Health Information for Caregivers and Families* by Charlotte M. Hendricks. Published by Redleaf Press. www.redleafpress.org.

Healthy Foods

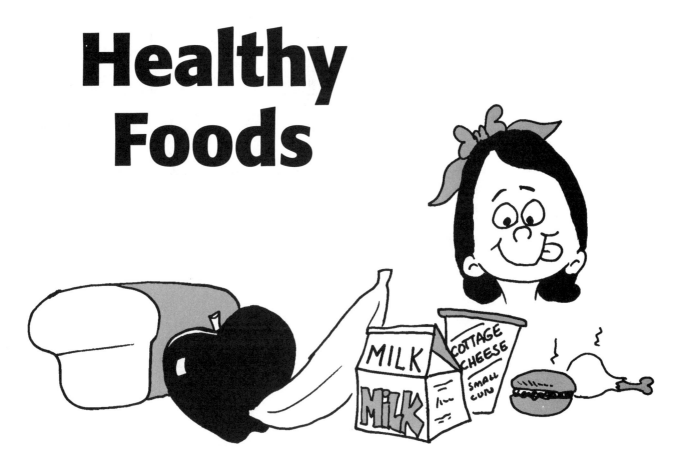

Children need a variety of foods each day.

Milk, cheese, eggs, yogurt, and lean meats are good sources of protein.

Vegetables, fruits, breads, oatmeal, grits, cereal, and rice contain vitamins and minerals needed for strong, healthy bodies.

Whole milk is good for children 1 to 2 years of age. Reduced-fat milk is recommended for children 2 years and older.

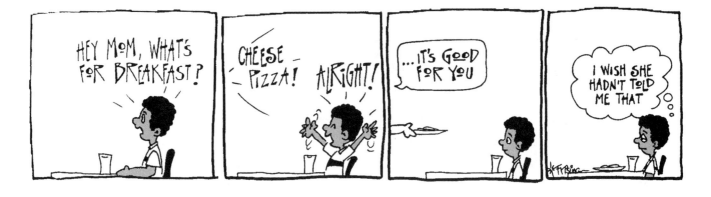

Healthy Foods

Children need three basic nutrients to grow strong and healthy—protein, carbohydrates, and fats. By eating a variety of healthy foods, most children will get the vitamins and minerals they need.

Protein: Children should eat some protein every day. Milk, cheese, eggs, peanut butter, yogurt, and lean meats are good sources of protein. Bacon, sausage, bologna, and hot dogs are not as good because they have very little protein and a lot of fat.

Carbohydrates: Vegetables, fruits, bread, oatmeal, grits, rice, cereal, muffins, toast, and pancakes are great foods for children. These foods contain vitamins and minerals needed to be strong and healthy. They need to eat foods like these several times a day.

Fats: Young children need a small amount of fat in their diet to help their body and brain develop. Whole milk is good for children ages one to two years. Low-fat milk is recommended for children two years and older. If children are eating a variety of foods, including proteins and carbohydrates, they are probably getting enough fat to meet their needs.

Limit the amount of fatty foods and sweets that children eat, such as potato chips, fried foods, and cookies.

From *Hip on Health: Health Information for Caregivers and Families* by Charlotte M. Hendricks. Published by Redleaf Press. www.redleafpress.org.

Lunchtime

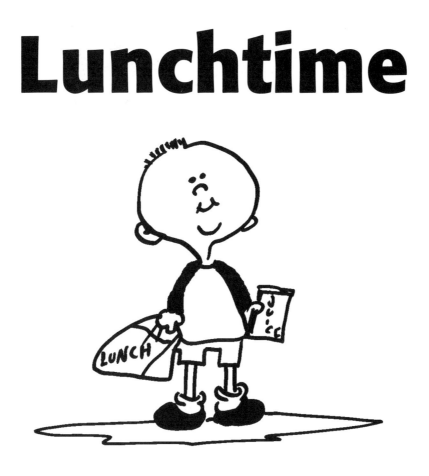

Packed lunches should be nutritious and safe. Whole wheat bread, bagels, rolls, pita pockets, English muffins, raisin bread, and flour tortillas are nutritious. Tuna and egg salads are packed with protein. Peanut butter on crackers is easy to eat.

Fruit cups and 100-percent juice boxes are healthy additions. Cheese, yogurt, pudding, and milk provide calcium.

Prevent foodborne illness by keeping foods cold. Use insulated lunch bags and freezable ice packs. Wash bags and freezer packs with warm soapy water each day.

From *Hip on Health: Health Information for Caregivers and Families* by Charlotte M. Hendricks. Published by Redleaf Press. www.redleafpress.org.

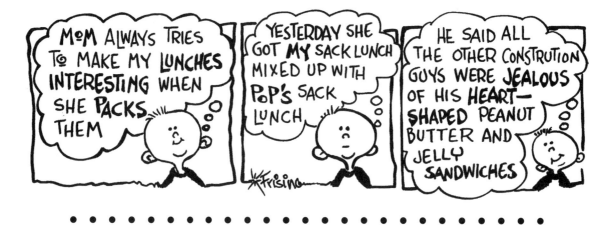

Lunchtime

Make sure packed lunches are nutritious and safe.

Use a variety of breads to make sandwiches interesting. Whole wheat bread, bagels, rolls, pita pockets, English muffins, raisin bread, and tortillas are nutritious. Pasta salad can be made with fun-shaped and colored pasta, such as small shells, wagon wheels, or ABCs.

Chicken, tuna, and egg salads are packed with protein. Lean cuts of ham, roast beef, or turkey are favorites with kids. Cheese or peanut butter on crackers is easy to eat.

Fruit cups and 100-percent juice boxes are healthy additions. Children get calcium by eating yogurt or pudding, and drinking milk or fortified juice.

Protect children from foodborne germs. Wash your hands before preparing or packing foods. Wash lunch containers and freezer packs with warm soapy water each day.

Keep cold foods cold and hot foods hot to prevent foodborne illness. Remember these tips:

✓ Use insulated lunch bags.

✓ Pack hot foods in insulated, sealed containers.

✓ Use freezable ice packs to keep food fresh and cool. Or freeze beverages and sandwiches the night before. They will thaw by lunchtime.

Pack love in the lunch bag! Hide special cards or pictures in the bag. Draw hearts to tell children how much you love them. Cut bread into fun surprise shapes with cookie cutters.

Mealtime

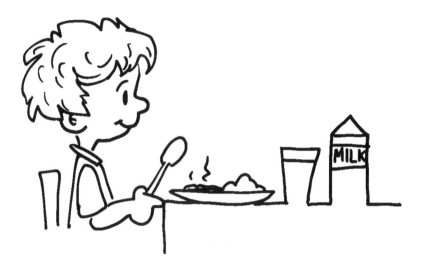

Children have small stomachs, so they may not eat much at a time. Instead, they need to eat often—about every three hours.

Give children a variety of foods, such as fruits and vegetables, cereals and bread, milk, cheese, and lean meats. It is okay for children to eat sweets occasionally if they also are eating other, healthier foods.

Offer water and milk to children to drink. Limit sweetened beverages, such as soda, tea, and fruit-flavored drinks.

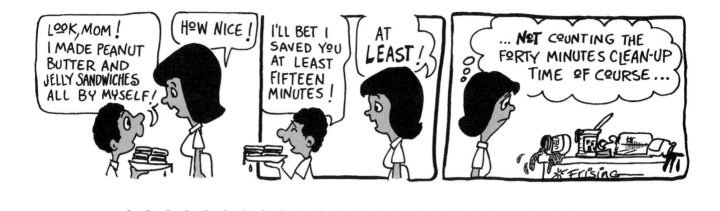

Mealtime

Children need breakfast to get through their busy mornings. After all, it has been ten or twelve hours since their last meal. Skipping breakfast can mean a growling tummy or a grumpy child. This can make it hard to do well in school.

Young children need to eat about every three hours, so give them small snacks between meals. Choose nutritious foods, such as fruit and cheese, peanut butter and crackers with milk, or half a sandwich with juice.

Young children need small servings of food (about ¼ cup per serving). Do not force them to eat everything on their plates. If children are served large portions of food and encouraged to eat it all, they may become overweight or learn to dislike certain foods.

Some children are picky eaters. Help prevent this by giving toddlers nutritious foods when they begin eating solid foods rather than sweets and candy.

Encourage children to try new foods. If they say they do not like a food, wait a few days and try that food again or prepare it a different way. Children will probably learn to like most foods, but you may need to serve a food twenty times before they like it! It is okay if there are some foods they will not eat.

Children may enjoy these meals or snacks:

✓ cheese pizza and juice

✓ fruit yogurt with dry cereal on top

✓ banana and peanut butter sandwich and juice

✓ cheese toast with a raisin face on top

✓ pancakes and eggs and milk

From *Hip on Health: Health Information for Caregivers and Families* by Charlotte M. Hendricks. Published by Redleaf Press. www.redleafpress.org.

Picky Eaters

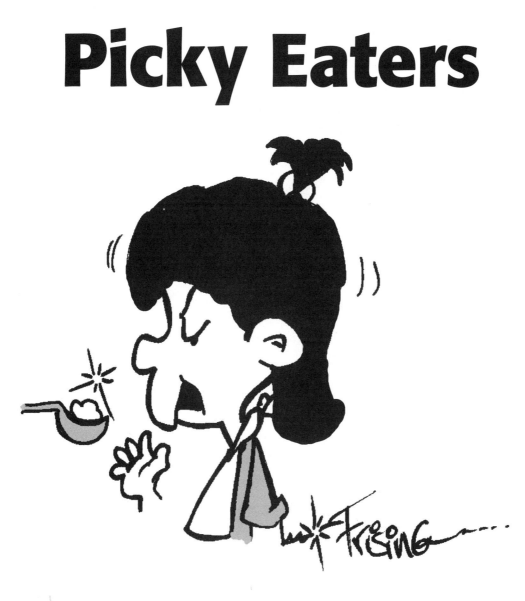

Many children have favorite foods. They may love a food one day and dislike it the next. It is okay if they occasionally do not eat a meal or if they want a specific food all week.

Children need a variety of foods. Encourage them to eat foods of different colors, shapes, textures, and flavors.

From *Hip on Health: Health Information for Caregivers and Families* by Charlotte M. Hendricks. Published by Redleaf Press. www.redleafpress.org.

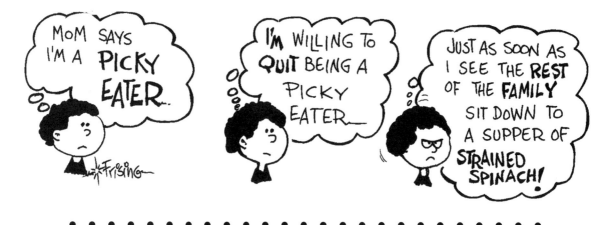

Picky Eaters

Many children have favorite foods. They may want a specific food, such as a peanut butter and jelly sandwich or macaroni and cheese, for every meal. Or they may insist on the same breakfast food for a month.

Children often change their minds about food. One day they may love a food, and the next day they may refuse to eat it.

Do not let food cause tension between you and children. It is okay if they occasionally do not eat a meal or if they prefer the same food for a week. Children do not have to eat every food that is offered.

As long as they are eating a variety of foods, they they are likely to receive the nutrients needed for healthy growth and development. For example, many fruits and vegetables have the same nutrients. Offer a few different foods at each meal. There is usually something picky eaters want to eat. Encourage children to eat foods of different colors, shapes, textures, and flavors.

With patience and a little planning, you may get even the pickiest eater to try new foods. Here are ways to encourage healthy eating:

✓ Add nutritious ingredients to favorite foods—for example, cut fruits or shredded vegetables in muffins.

✓ Let children help prepare foods.

✓ Offer healthy choices and encourage children to pick the ones they prefer.

✓ Try to include at least one food you know each child likes in every meal.

✓ Provide nutritious snack foods between meals. Avoid sweetened beverages and sugary snacks.

From *Hip on Health: Health Information for Caregivers and Families* by Charlotte M. Hendricks. Published by Redleaf Press. www.redleafpress.org.

Snacktime

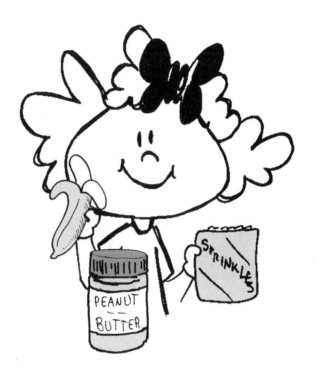

Snacks help provide the energy children need to make it through the day. Provide good-tasting and good-for-you foods at snacktime.

Avoid snacks that are high in sugar, salt, and fat.

Create special snacks—for example, a banana smeared with a little peanut butter and colorful sprinkles on top!

From *Hip on Health: Health Information for Caregivers and Families* by Charlotte M. Hendricks. Published by Redleaf Press. www.redleafpress.org.

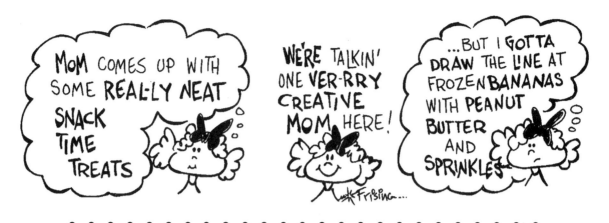

Snacktime

Snacks are important for young children. They have small tummies and need to eat every three to four hours. Between-meal snacks provide the energy they need to make it through the day.

Promote children's growth and development by offering good-tasting and good-for-you foods.

Here are some ideas for easy, nutritious snacks:

✓ fresh fruit, applesauce, and fruit cups

✓ shredded fresh veggies with low-fat dressing

✓ low-fat yogurt and pudding

✓ minipretzels, breadsticks, and rice cakes

✓ low-fat, low-sugar cereal

✓ granola bars, graham crackers, and whole-wheat crackers

Make ordinary foods more fun. Try frozen fruit juice on a stick or frozen bananas. Make special snacks like bananas smeared with a little peanut butter or yogurt and sprinkles on top.

Remember, young children can easily choke on foods that are hard, round, tough, slippery, or sticky. Make sure snack foods are safe foods!

Bath Time Safety

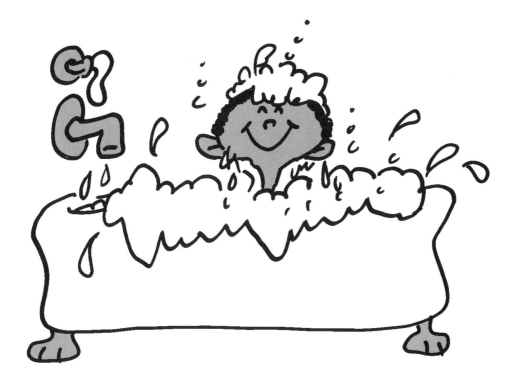

Splashing, bath toys, and your gentle touch make bath time a fun activity. However, children can be injured by burns, falls, or drowning.

Never leave children under 6 years alone in a bathtub. They can drown in just a few inches of water. Drowning usually occurs quickly and silently—for example, while you answer the phone. Never leave a young child alone in the tub for even a second!

From *Hip on Health: Health Information for Caregivers and Families* by Charlotte M. Hendricks. Published by Redleaf Press. www.redleafpress.org.

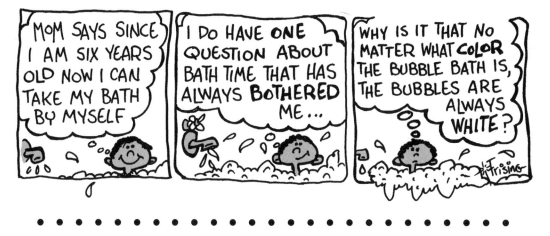

Bath Time Safety

Bath time can be fun for children. Splashing, bath toys, and your gentle touch make it a favorite activity. But children can be injured during bath time from burns, falls, or drowning.

Never leave children under six years alone in the bathtub! They can drown in just a few inches of water. Drowning usually occurs quickly and silently—for example, while you answer the phone. Children lose consciousness in two minutes and can sustain brain damage or death in four to six minutes. Never leave young children alone in a bathtub for even a second!

Baby bath seats and rings are bathing aids—they are not safety devices. Infants should always be within adult reach. If children bathe together, do not make older children responsible for younger sisters or brothers. An adult should always supervise.

Children have very tender skin and can be seriously burned in bath water. Lower the thermostat on your hot water heater to 120°F. Teach children to keep their hands away from the handles and spigots. Enclose the spout with a soft cover to help prevent burns and injuries caused by bumping into it.

Remove adult bathing items, such as shampoo or razors, from children's bathing area. Unplug electric appliances, such as hair dryers, immediately after use.

Clean up spills and dry children's feet after bathing to prevent slips.

Burns

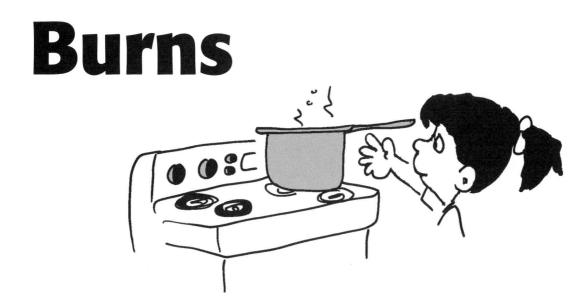

Children can be burned by hot liquids, fire, and hot surfaces. They may not know when something is hot. Help prevent burns by doing the following:

- Lower your hot water heater to 120°F.

- Do not smoke or drink hot liquids while holding a child.

- Keep cigarettes, matches, and lighters out of children's reach.

- Do not place heaters near children's play areas.

- Keep children away from open fireplaces and cooking grills.

- Check food temperatures, especially those of microwaved foods.

From *Hip on Health: Health Information for Caregivers and Families* by Charlotte M. Hendricks. Published by Redleaf Press. www.redleafpress.org.

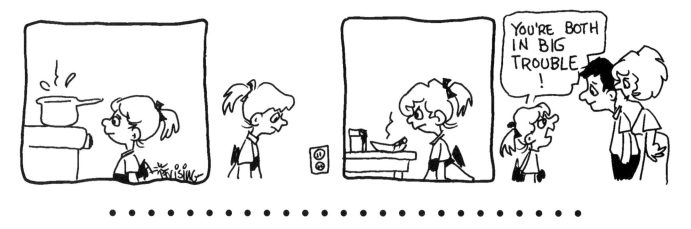

Burns

Burns can cause scars, permanent damage, or death. Even a small burn on a young child can be serious. If a child is burned, cool the burn with lots of cold running water. Do *not* use butter or ointment. Here are ways to prevent burns:

✓ Lower the thermostat on your hot water heater to 120°F. Children can become seriously burned in less than five seconds if the water is too hot.

✓ Keep children away from the stove while you are cooking. Turn pot handles toward the back of the stove. Never put crock pots, deep fryers, and hot foods where children can reach them. Make sure cords for cooking appliances are also out of reach.

✓ Stir microwaved food and feel how hot it is before serving. Microwaved foods can have hot spots in the center of the food.

✓ Do not heat infant formula in the microwave.

✓ Put safety covers over unused electrical outlets. Teach children not to play with cords or to touch electrical outlets. Throw away electrical cords with frayed wires.

✓ Do not let children play near heaters, fireplaces, or stoves. Do not place cribs or playpens near heaters, radiators, fireplaces, or stoves.

✓ Keep matches, cigarette lighters, and cigarettes away from children.

From *Hip on Health: Health Information for Caregivers and Families* by Charlotte M. Hendricks. Published by Redleaf Press. www.redleafpress.org.

Choking

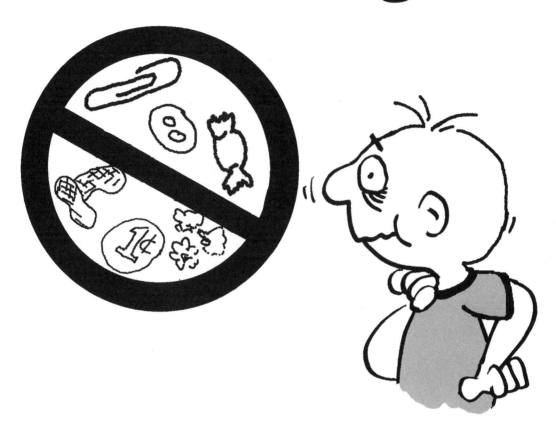

Small, round, and hard foods can cause choking. Hot dogs, popcorn, nuts, hard candies, and bubble gum are some of the most dangerous foods.

Children can choke on popped or uninflated balloons. Small objects, such as paper clips, buttons, and coins, can also cause choking.

Do not let children run and play with anything in their mouths.

From *Hip on Health: Health Information for Caregivers and Families* by Charlotte M. Hendricks. Published by Redleaf Press. www.redleafpress.org.

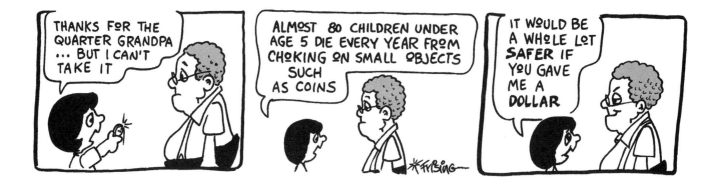

Choking

Approximately eighty children age five and under die of choking every year. Choking can usually be prevented.

When children start crawling and walking, check the areas they use carefully for small objects. Look under couch cushions and under furniture and all over floors for rubber bands, paper clips, safety pins, and other small objects. If children are younger than four years old, be sure their toys do not have small or broken parts.

Children can choke on coins, jacks, marbles, and other small objects. Teach them to keep objects like pins, coins, and caps from ink pens out of their mouths. Latex balloons are dangerous! If a child inhales a piece of balloon,

it can cover the windpipe, and you may not be able to remove it.

Young children can choke on foods that are slippery, hard, or round, such as nuts, hard candy, ice, and popcorn. Hot dogs and grapes are dangerous because they are round and because the skin of the hot dog or grape can block the child's windpipe. Skin these foods and cut them into small pieces. Sticky foods, such as a spoonful of peanut butter or a handful of raisins, also can cause choking.

Teach children to chew food carefully. Do not allow them to run or jump while eating food, candy, or chewing gum. Do not allow children walk or run with other objects in their mouths.

From *Hip on Health: Health Information for Caregivers and Families* by Charlotte M. Hendricks. Published by Redleaf Press. www.redleafpress.org.

Fire Safety

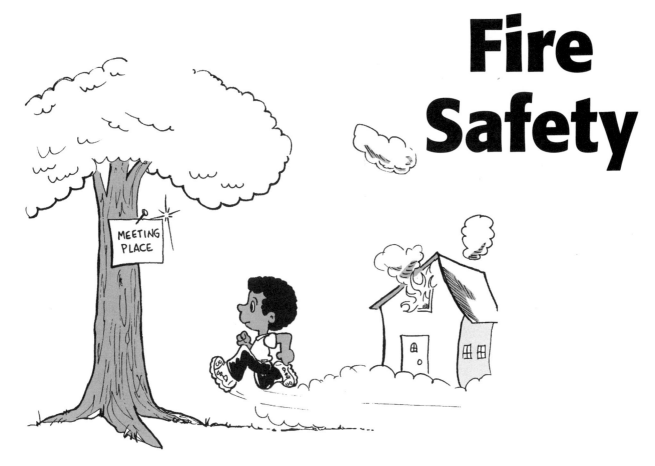

Most children like to watch fires. They may play with matches or lighters when adults are not watching them. Keep matches and lighters out of their reach.

Teach children what to do in case of fire:

- Get out fast!

- "Get low and go!" if there is smoke.

- "Stop, drop, and roll" if your clothes catch on fire.

- Go to the meeting place outside.

From *Hip on Health: Health Information for Caregivers and Families* by Charlotte M. Hendricks. Published by Redleaf Press. www.redleafpress.org.

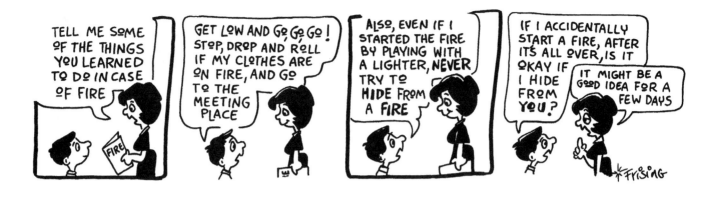

Fire Safety

Fire and burns are leading causes of death for young children. Most children would not know what to do if they smelled smoke or saw fire. Some children try to hide from a fire, especially if they started it by playing with matches or lighters.

In just thirty seconds, a small flame from a dropped match can become a fire burning out of control. Smoke and heat are deadly. The air temperature can reach 600°F at adult eye level and up to 1,500°F near a ceiling. If a smoke detector goes off two minutes after a fire starts, you may have less than two minutes to get out of the house!

Install smoke detectors on the ceiling or high on the wall of each floor in your house. Place smoke detectors close to bedrooms and at the top of stairs. Test them every month.

Follow the manufacturer's instructions on the smoke detector. Change batteries as recommended, usually twice each year. Pick a date that is easy to remember, such as when daylight saving time changes. Replace smoke detectors every ten years.

Teach children what to do if there is a fire in your home or building. No matter what caused the fire, just get out and be safe! Here are some things young children can learn:

- ✓ Get out of the house fast!

- ✓ "Get low and go!" when there is smoke in the building.

- ✓ Know emergency exits from bedrooms. Practice opening a locked window and pushing out a screen. If the window is a few feet above the ground, show them how to hang from their hands and drop to the ground.

- ✓ "Stop, drop, and roll" if your clothes catch on fire.

- ✓ Know a safe meeting place outside where everyone should go.

From *Hip on Health: Health Information for Caregivers and Families* by Charlotte M. Hendricks. Published by Redleaf Press. www.redleafpress.org.

Gun Safety

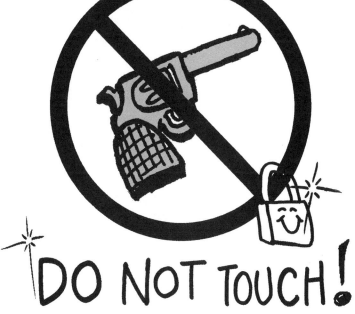

Every year children die from gunshot wounds.

The best way to prevent injury and death from guns is to make sure guns are not accessible to children.

Make sure gun safety rules are followed in your home and in other homes they visit.

Teach children "Do not touch! Go tell an adult!" if they find a gun.

From *Hip on Health: Health Information for Caregivers and Families* by Charlotte M. Hendricks. Published by Redleaf Press. www.redleafpress.org.

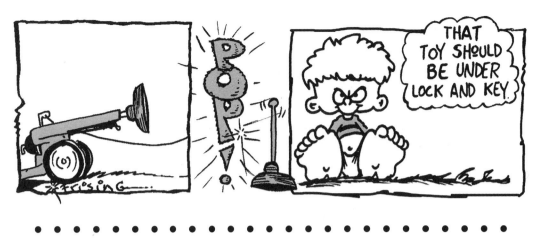

Gun Safety

Every year, children die from gunshot wounds. Children cannot always tell the difference between toy guns and real weapons. The best way to prevent injury and death from firearms is to avoid keeping guns in areas accessible to children and avoid exposing children to households where guns are kept.

Protect children by ensuring that gun safety rules are followed in your own home and in homes where children may visit. Guns should be unloaded and stored in a locked cabinet. Ammunition should also be stored in locked containers separate from guns.

Anyone who handles or owns guns should take a gun safety course and always practice gun safety. Teach children that guns are not toys and should never be played with.

Talk with children about what to do if they find a gun or see someone with a gun:

✓ Stop! Do not touch.

✓ Get away.

✓ Tell a trusted adult.

From *Hip on Health: Health Information for Caregivers and Families* by Charlotte M. Hendricks. Published by Redleaf Press. www.redleafpress.org.

Indoor Safety

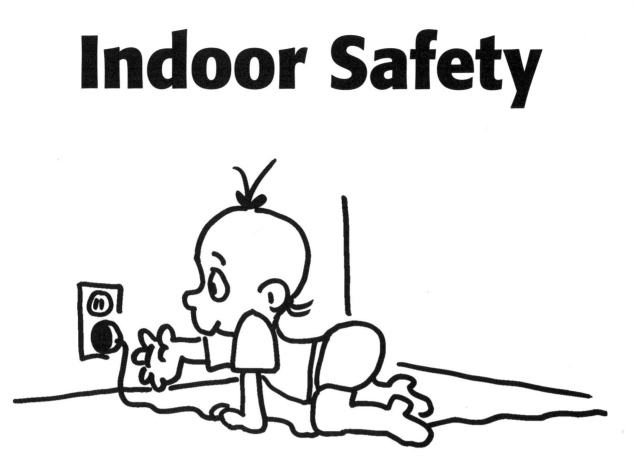

Keep poisons and medicines out of children's sight and out of reach. Check under sinks, in closets, and in garages for poisonous substances. Keep medicines in child-resistant containers.

Store knives, scissors, and sharp objects out of children's reach.

Store guns and bullets in locked cabinets. Guns should be unloaded.

Keep matches, lighters, and cigarettes out of children's reach.

Cover unused electrical outlets with safety caps.

From *Hip on Health: Health Information for Caregivers and Families* by Charlotte M. Hendricks. Published by Redleaf Press. www.redleafpress.org.

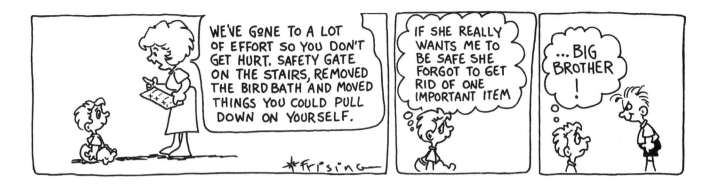

Indoor Safety

You can make your home safer and prevent injury to children by doing the following:

✓ Check under sinks, in closets, and in garages for poisonous substances like dishwashing and laundry soaps, cleaner, paint thinner, and insecticide. Keep poisons out of children's sight and out of reach.

✓ Keep all medicines, including vitamins, out of sight, out of reach, and in child-resistant containers.

✓ Store knives, scissors, and sharp objects out of children's reach.

✓ Store guns and bullets in locked cabinets. Guns should be unloaded.

✓ Keep matches, lighters, and cigarettes out of children's reach.

✓ Prevent strangulation by tying up or using a clothespin to keep curtain and blind cords out of reach.

✓ Keep small objects that can cause choking away from infants and toddlers.

✓ Prevent falls by clearing stairways of toys and other objects. Remove throw rugs.

✓ Bolt bookshelves and cabinets securely to walls so children cannot climb them. Be sure heavy objects, such as televisions, cannot fall off shelves.

✓ Cover unused electrical outlets with safety caps.

From *Hip on Health: Health Information for Caregivers and Families* by Charlotte M. Hendricks. Published by Redleaf Press. www.redleafpress.org.

Lead Poisoning

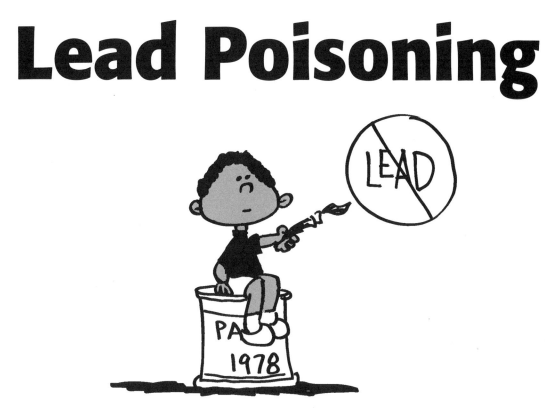

Lead poisoning can affect children's growth, damage their kidneys, impair their hearing, cause vomiting and headaches, and impair learning and cause behavioral problems.

You can help prevent lead poisoning:

- Repaint old walls, windowsills, and furniture.

- Wash children's hands often.

- Clean floors, window frames, windowsills, and other surfaces.

- Plant grass or other ground cover in children's play areas.

From *Hip on Health: Health Information for Caregivers and Families* by Charlotte M. Hendricks. Published by Redleaf Press. www.redleafpress.org.

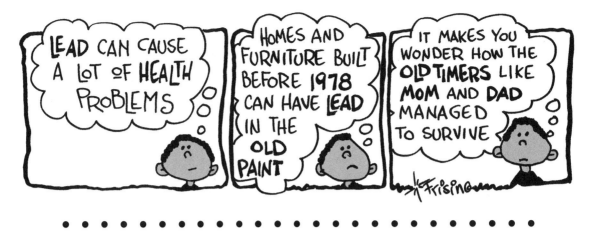

Lead Poisoning

Lead is a highly toxic metal. If children eat or breathe lead dust, it can affect their growth. Lead can also damage kidneys, impair hearing, cause vomiting, headaches, and learning and behavioral problems.

Homes and furniture built before 1978 may have old paint that contains lead. Metal water pipes and solder may contain lead. Soil can be contaminated with lead from diesel, gasoline, and car exhaust. Products used in making pottery or stained glass, fishing weights, and reloading ammunition may contain lead. Imported pottery often contains lead.

Here are some ways to help prevent lead poisoning:

✓ Clean up paint chips. Repaint old walls and furniture.

✓ Wash children's hands before they eat.

✓ Clean floors, window frames, windowsills, and other surfaces with warm water and household cleaner.

✓ Be sure children eat nutritious meals and snacks because well-nourished children are at less risk from lead poisoning.

✓ Cover dirt contaminated by vehicle exhaust or fuel with grass or other ground cover in children's play areas.

✓ Let tap water run several seconds before getting water for drinking or cooking.

✓ Use appropriate precautions when remodeling houses or facilities built before 1978.

From *Hip on Health: Health Information for Caregivers and Families* by Charlotte M. Hendricks. Published by Redleaf Press. www.redleafpress.org.

Poisons

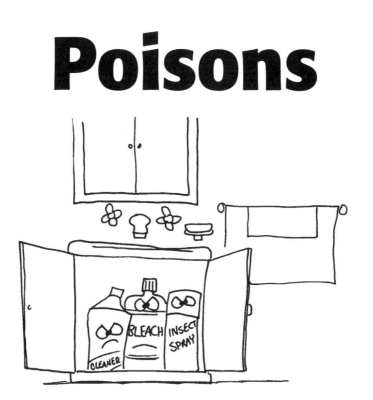

Look under sinks and in cabinets for cleaners, insect sprays, and other poisons.

Products such as dishwasher detergent, laundry detergent, and toilet cleaner can burn inside children's mouths, throats, and stomachs. Children can have serious injuries or die within minutes.

Child-resistant latches are not enough. Many children can open these latches. Keep cleaning supplies and other poisons out of children's sight and reach.

If children swallow or breathe a poison, call the Poison Control Center *immediately* at 1-800-222-1222.

From *Hip on Health: Health Information for Caregivers and Families* by Charlotte M. Hendricks. Published by Redleaf Press. www.redleafpress.org.

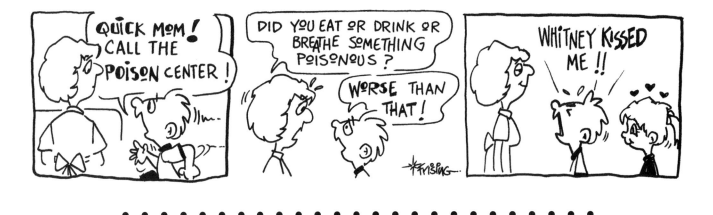

Poison

Cleaning supplies, bleach, makeup, medicine, shampoo, and other products found in the house can be poisonous if swallowed, breathed, or splashed on skin or in eyes.

Keep cleaning supplies away from children. Products such as dishwasher detergent, laundry detergent, and toilet cleaner can burn the insides of their mouths, throats, airways, and stomachs. Do not store cleaning supplies under sinks or in cabinets, even with safety latches. Many children can open these latches. Keep cleaning products in locked cabinets out of children's sight and reach.

Poisons can be found in many places. For example, many people keep medicine in their purses or backpacks. Keep all medicines out of children's sight and reach.

Poisoning can occur quickly. Children can sustain serious injuries or die within minutes. Children can swallow cleaner left on a table in just seconds. Detergent pods for laundry or dishwashers are attractive to children but can be deadly if eaten. Close containers and put them away immediately after use. Never put poisonous substances in beverage or food containers.

Many plants are poisonous. Chewing the leaves of some plants can cause swelling in the mouth and breathing problems. Many mushrooms are poisonous. Azalea, aloe, and lily of the valley are just a few of the many poisonous plants. Teach children to keep plants out of their mouths.

If children swallow or breathe something that could make them sick, call the **Poison Control Center** *immediately* at **1-800-222-1222**. Identify what they have swallowed or breathed. You will be told what to do.

**Poison Control Center
1-800-222-1222**

From *Hip on Health: Health Information for Caregivers and Families* by Charlotte M. Hendricks. Published by Redleaf Press. www.redleafpress.org.

Suffocation and Strangulation

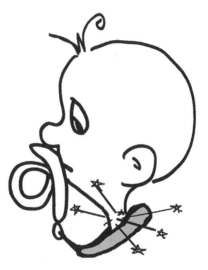

Children can strangle on loose cords and strings. Never tie necklaces or pacifiers around their necks. Remove drawstrings from clothing.

When infants can pull themselves up, remove crib mobiles and hanging toys that they can reach.

Keep window blind cords out of reach by tying them or using clothespins to hold them up.

Keep dry-cleaning bags and other plastic bags out of children's reach.

From *Hip on Health: Health Information for Caregivers and Families* by Charlotte M. Hendricks. Published by Redleaf Press. www.redleafpress.org.

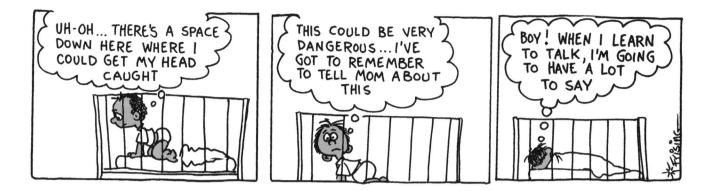

Suffocation and Strangulation

Protect infants from suffocation and strangulation.

- ✓ Do not lay infants on water beds, soft blankets, pillows, and sofas where they can be trapped between the cushions.

- ✓ Infants should not sleep in the same bed with adults or other children. The larger person may roll over on the infant while asleep.

- ✓ Old cribs can be dangerous. Cutouts in headboards can trap children's heads. Corner posts can catch on clothing and cause children to strangle. Post tops should be cut even with headboards.

- ✓ Make sure mattresses fit tightly against all four sides of cribs.

- ✓ Fitted crib sheets should be large enough to completely cover mattresses. Be sure they cannot slip off mattresses and wrap around infants.

- ✓ Spaces between crib slats should be no more than 2³⁄₈ inches. Spaces wider than this can trap infants' heads.

- ✓ When infants can pull themselves up, remove crib gyms, mobiles, and hanging toys that they can reach.

Children can strangle on loose cords and strings.

- ✓ Never tie necklaces or pacifiers around children's necks.

- ✓ Window blind cords should be out of children's reach. Tie them up or use clothespins to hold them high.

- ✓ Remove drawstrings from children's clothing. Drawstrings can catch on play equipment, fences, or other objects and cause strangulation.

Never leave dry-cleaning or other plastic bags where children can reach them.

From *Hip on Health: Health Information for Caregivers and Families* by Charlotte M. Hendricks. Published by Redleaf Press. www.redleafpress.org.

Toy Safety

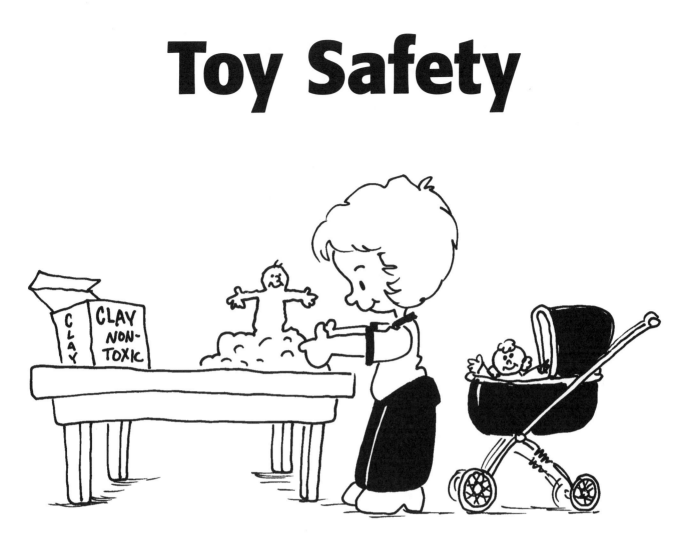

Read toy instructions before giving the toys to children to play with. Check the recommended ages listed on the package to see if they are appropriate for the children.

Children under four years old should not play with toys with small parts. They can choke on small pieces.

Be sure all painted toys, paints, crayons, glues, and modeling clay are labeled "nontoxic."

From *Hip on Health: Health Information for Caregivers and Families* by Charlotte M. Hendricks. Published by Redleaf Press. www.redleafpress.org.

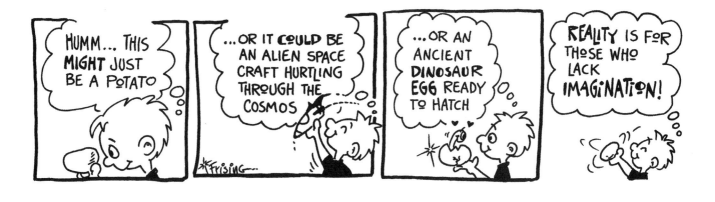

Toy Safety

Children have great imaginations and can create ways to play with almost anything. Often they have more fun with pots and pans than with expensive toys.

The best toys allow children to imagine and create ways to use them. Blocks, cars and trucks, and dolls allow children to imagine entire worlds. Art supplies like crayons, paints, modeling clay, glue, and scissors promote creativity.

When choosing toys and materials, be sure they are safe for children. Always read the instructions. Most toys and games have recommended ages printed on the package. Toys recommended for older children may not be safe for younger children.

Toys for children under four years old should not have small parts that can cause choking. If you have also have toys for older children, be sure young children do not get hurt by these toys.

Be sure all paints, markers, modeling clay, and painted toys are labeled "nontoxic." Inspect toys for sharp edges or broken parts.

Some items are dangerous for children. Pellet and BB guns, bow and arrows, darts, and knives are not toys. Children can seriously injure themselves or others with these.

From *Hip on Health: Health Information for Caregivers and Families* by Charlotte M. Hendricks. Published by Redleaf Press. www.redleafpress.org.

Toy Safety– Infants

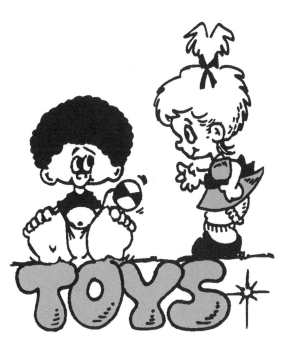

Mobiles and crib toys should be securely fastened in place and out of infants' reach. Remove these toys from the crib when infants are able to push up on their hands and knees.

Do not put stuffed animals or pillows in infants' cribs.

Think big for infant toys. Rattles and teething toys should be indestructible and pliable, and large to prevent choking.

From *Hip on Health: Health Information for Caregivers and Families* by Charlotte M. Hendricks. Published by Redleaf Press. www.redleafpress.org.

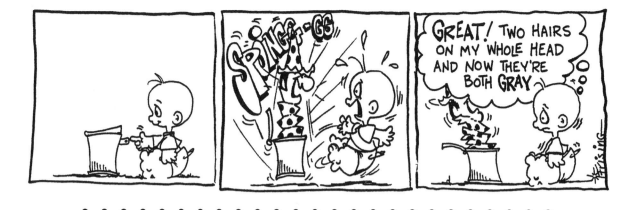

Toy Safety—Infants

Keep mobiles and crib toys out of infants' reach! Infants can become tangled in the cords used to attach mobiles or crib gyms, causing strangulation. Children can pull crib toys down on themselves, causing injury.

Crib toys should be securely fastened in place and out of infants' reach. Remove toys from cribs when infants are able to push up on their hands and knees (at about five months).

Check stuffed toys carefully. Make sure tails and ears are sewn on securely and seams are reinforced. Check for buttons, yarn, ribbon, or other parts that children can pull off. Do not put stuffed animals or pillows in infants' cribs. These can cause suffocation.

Think big for infants' toys. Infants put things in their mouths, so keep small objects out of reach. Check toys for small parts, such as noise-making squeakers, which can fall out and cause choking. Rattles and teething toys should be indestructible and pliable, and large to prevent choking.

Measure toys for safety by trying to fit them inside a choking tube. Use an empty toilet paper roll to measure toys' choking potential. If a toy fits inside the tube, it is too small for children to have.

Avoid latex balloons! These are one of the leading causes of choking deaths. Avoid toys with strings longer than twelve inches.

Children's toy boxes should have sturdy hinges, well-supported lids that do not slam shut, and ventilation holes in case children crawl inside.

From *Hip on Health: Health Information for Caregivers and Families* by Charlotte M. Hendricks. Published by Redleaf Press. www.redleafpress.org.

Toy Safety— Toddlers

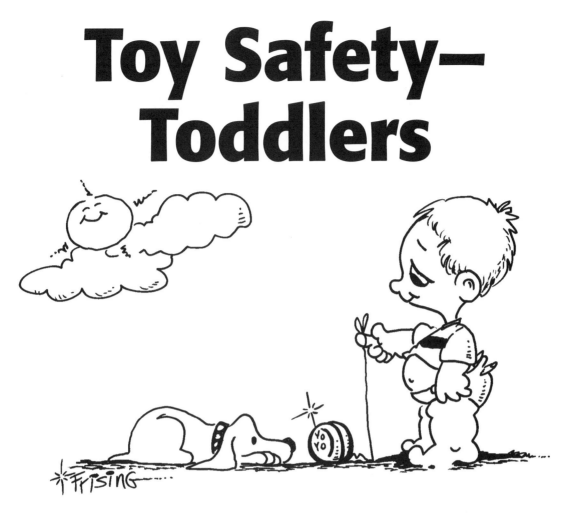

The first three years of life are an important learning period. Choose toys that allow children to explore and have safe fun:

- Follow recommended age levels and warnings on toy packages.

- Avoid toys with small parts.

- Avoid toys with long cords and strings.

- Choose art and craft items labeled "nontoxic."

From *Hip on Health: Health Information for Caregivers and Families* by Charlotte M. Hendricks. Published by Redleaf Press. www.redleafpress.org.

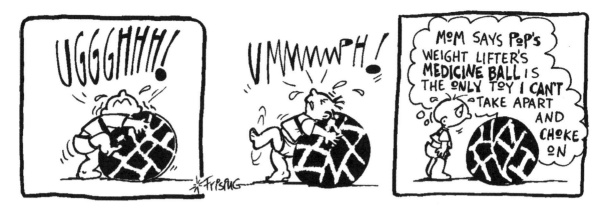

Toy Safety—Toddlers

The first three years of life are an important learning period. Choose toys that allow children to explore and have fun.

Blocks in various shapes and sizes encourage pretend play. Blocks can be made of wood, cardboard, or soft materials. Include other toys, such as trucks, cars, and wagons, which toddlers can dump and fill with blocks. Adding toy animals and people encourages children to use their imaginations.

Toys should be safe and appropriate for children's ages and abilities:

✓ Follow recommended age levels and warnings on toy packages.

✓ Avoid toys with small parts.

✓ Check dolls and stuffed animals for small parts (buttons, eyes, noses) that could be pulled off.

✓ Choose art and craft items labeled "nontoxic."

✓ Wash toys frequently.

Toddlers put things in their mouths, so toys should be large to prevent choking. You can measure a toy by trying to fit it inside a choking tube. An empty toilet paper roll can measure toys' choking potential. If a toy fits inside the tube, then it is too small for children to have.

Avoid toys with long cords or strings. Keep latex balloons away from toddlers.

From *Hip on Health: Health Information for Caregivers and Families* by Charlotte M. Hendricks. Published by Redleaf Press. www.redleafpress.org.

Toy Safety– Preschool

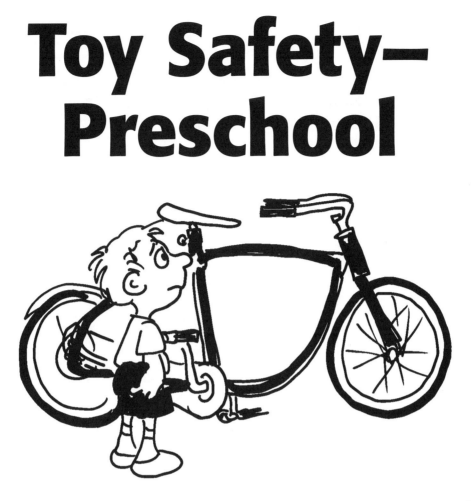

Make sure children's toys are safe. Follow age recommendations on the package.

Avoid these potentially dangerous toys:

- **motorized vehicles, such as scooters or go-carts**

- **toys that shoot projectiles**

- **toys that make loud noises**

- **chemistry sets or toys with toxic materials**

From *Hip on Health: Health Information for Caregivers and Families* by Charlotte M. Hendricks. Published by Redleaf Press. www.redleafpress.org.

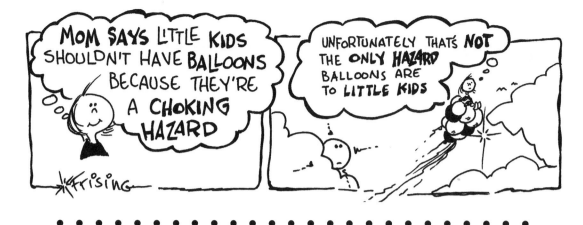

Toy Safety—Preschool

Most preschoolers are ready for toys that develop thinking and fine-motor skills. Simple puzzles, board games, peg boards, small connecting blocks, and lacing cards are good choices.

Children enjoy wooden blocks. They can sort, pile, haul, and stack them to construct simple or intricate structures. Adding animals, small vehicles, rug or cloth scraps, empty paper towel tubes, or paper cups allows children to use blocks in a whole new way, thus extending their learning experience.

Choose wheeled toys that are well balanced, with wide wheels that have adequate tread. Riding toys should match the size of the children, allowing them to firmly grasp the handles and reach the foot pedals. Insist that children always wear properly fitted helmets!

Electrical toys require careful adult supervision. Teach children to respect electricity.

Consider the ages and abilities of the children who will play with the toys. Read and follow the age recommendations and warnings on the package. Choking is still a hazard for preschoolers, so supervise them carefully. Here are some toys to avoid:

- ✓ latex balloons, which can cause choking

- ✓ motorized vehicles, such as scooters and go-carts

- ✓ toys that shoot projectiles, BB or pellet guns, dart games, and bows and arrows

- ✓ toys that make loud noises

- ✓ chemistry sets or toys with toxic materials

From *Hip on Health: Health Information for Caregivers and Families* by Charlotte M. Hendricks. Published by Redleaf Press. www.redleafpress.org.

Window Safety

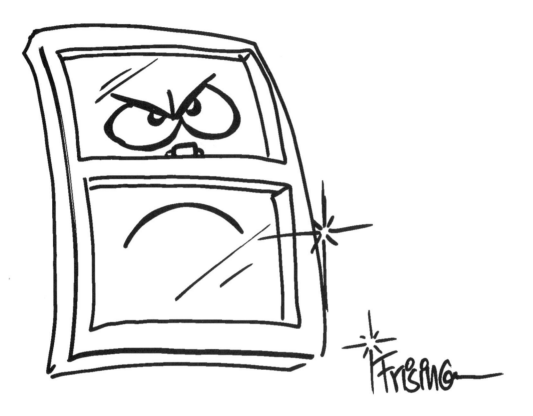

Each year, children are injured by falls from windows.

Place cribs, playpens, beds, chairs, and furniture away from windows. Window screens cannot prevent falls. Put sturdy barriers in front of low windows, such as child safety fencing.

Windows may be needed as escape routes in case of fire. Practice fire drills with children, including how to safely exit windows.

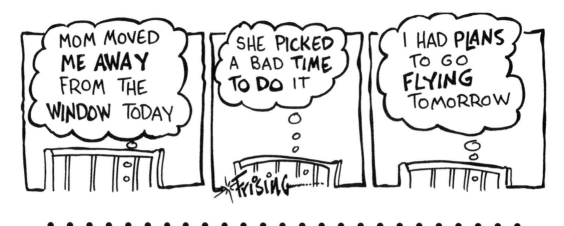

Window Safety

Falls from even first-floor windows can seriously injure or kill children. Falling through glass can cause serious injury. Children can be strangled if they become tangled in cords or window coverings.

Check every window and follow safety tips:

✓ Position cribs, playpens, beds, and furniture away from windows.

✓ Put sturdy barriers in front of low windows, such as child safety fencing. Window screens cannot prevent children from falling out.

✓ Make sure windows in play rooms, bedrooms, and other unsupervised areas cannot be easily opened by young children.

✓ Plant soft shrubs or grass under windows. If falls occur, softer landing surfaces may reduce the risk of serious injuries.

✓ Keep window cords out of children's reach. Use clips or clothespins to hold cords high. Anchor continuous-loop cords to floors or walls.

Children can be injured by running into glass doors. Make doors more visible by taping children's artwork to doors. Avoid vinyl or gel decorations because very young children may put them in their mouths.

Windows may be needed as escape routes in case of fire, so make sure they can open. They should not be painted or nailed shut. Window guards, security bars, grilles, and grates must have release mechanisms. Practice fire drills with children, including how to safely exit windows.

From *Hip on Health: Health Information for Caregivers and Families* by Charlotte M. Hendricks. Published by Redleaf Press. www.redleafpress.org.

Heat Illness

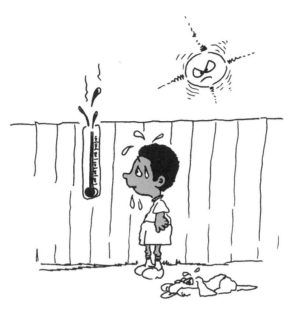

Children can become sick if they get too hot. Here are ways to help them enjoy warm weather safely:

- **Give children plenty of fluids to drink, especially water.**

- **Let children play indoors or in the shade during the hottest part of the day.**

- **Be sure children have shady play areas.**

- **Dress children in comfortable, cool clothes.**

***Never* leave children in parked vehicles during hot weather. Even with the windows open, vehicles can become dangerously hot in a few minutes.**

From *Hip on Health: Health Information for Caregivers and Families* by Charlotte M. Hendricks. Published by Redleaf Press. www.redleafpress.org.

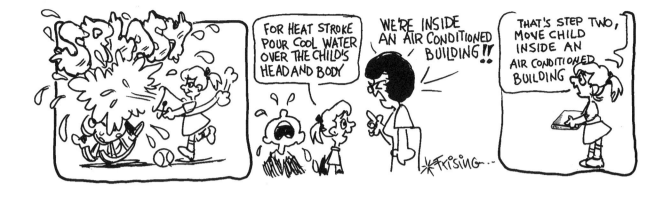

Heat Illness

Too much heat and sun can be dangerous, especially for children. *Never* leave them in parked vehicles, even for a few minutes. Even with the windows open, the temperature inside vehicles can reach 120°F or higher in a few minutes.

Dehydration occurs when children do not drink enough water or fluid. Children who are dehydrated may have dry skin and mouth, sunken eyes, or not use the bathroom within six hours. Help prevent dehydration by giving children plenty of water and fluids to drink.

Heat exhaustion can occur when children become too hot, lose fluid by sweating, and do not drink enough water. They may become weak, dizzy, or confused, suffer nausea or muscle cramps, and may faint. Get them to a cool place immediately! If they are awake, give sips of cool water or juice. If they do not feel better in a few minutes, or if their temperature goes up (fever), call emergency help (911)!

Heatstroke causes children's body temperature to rise very high, very fast. Signs of heatstroke include hot, red and dry skin, rapid heartbeat, and high temperature. Children may have breathing problems, headache, confusion, dizziness, or convulsions.

Heatstroke is life threatening! You must cool children fast! Pour lots of cool water over their heads and bodies, being careful not to get water in their noses or mouths. Place cold packs in their armpits and between their legs. Move them into an air-conditioned building and call emergency help (911)! If they are awake, give them sips of cool water.

From *Hip on Health: Health Information for Caregivers and Families* by Charlotte M. Hendricks. Published by Redleaf Press. www.redleafpress.org.

Helmets and Safety

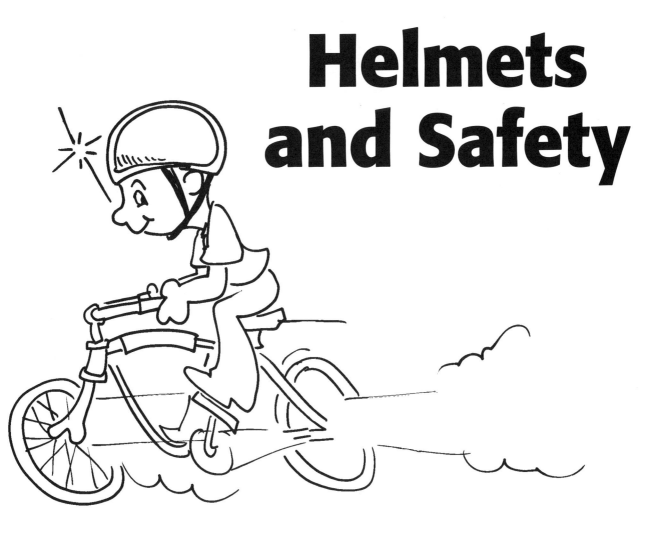

Children and adults should wear helmets when on bikes, skateboards, ice skates, roller skates, or in-line skates.

Helmets help prevent head injuries, as well as broken noses, cut faces, and lost teeth.

Helmets should fit snugly, but not tightly. Be sure they are comfortable and cover the forehead.

Remember—even professionals wear helmets!

From *Hip on Health: Health Information for Caregivers and Families* by Charlotte M. Hendricks. Published by Redleaf Press. www.redleafpress.org.

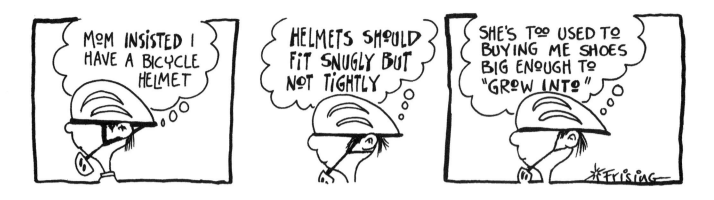

Helmets and Safety

Bicycle-related injuries can happen even when children are careful. For example, they can crash under the following circumstances:

✓ a driver does not see the child or the child rides in front of a vehicle

✓ a vehicle suddenly comes out of a side street or driveway

✓ a vehicle door opens as the child rides by

✓ the bike tire hits a rock, stick, or hole

✓ the child crashes into a stationary object, such as a mailbox

Children learning to ride bikes should not ride on streets with vehicles. Choose a level area away from traffic. Always supervise children. Teach them to watch for vehicles.

Make sure the bikes are the correct size. Children's feet should touch the ground when they are sitting on the bike. Young children need bikes with foot brakes rather than hand brakes.

Give children helmets with their first tricycle or bike. Insist that they always wear helmets when riding bikes or skateboards and when ice skating or in-line skating. Helmets helps prevent head injuries, as well as broken noses, cut faces, and lost teeth.

Helmets should have a label demonstrating Ansi, Snell, or CPSC approval. They should fit snugly, but not tightly. Position them to cover foreheads. Most helmets have foam pads and chin straps that can be changed to make them fit. Adjust helmets so they are comfortable and do not slide around.

From *Hip on Health: Health Information for Caregivers and Families* by Charlotte M. Hendricks. Published by Redleaf Press. www.redleafpress.org.

Hot Car

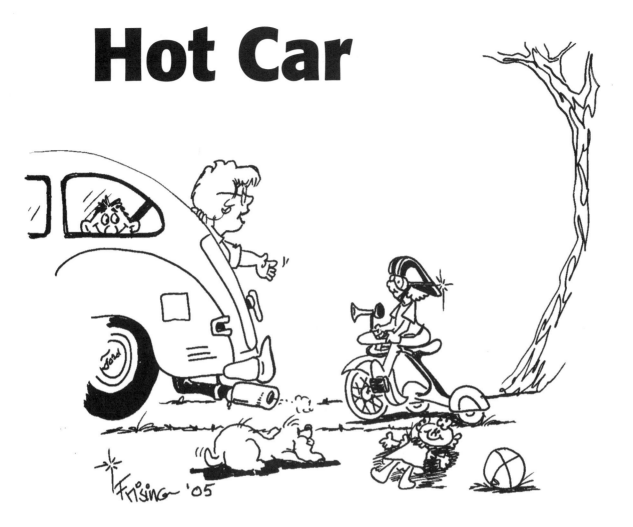

Never leave children alone in or around vehicles—not even for a minute. On a warm or sunny day, the temperature inside a vehicle can reach 120°F or higher in just a few minutes, even with the windows open.

Check the back seat! A child left in a hot car can suffer serious injury or death in less than an hour.

From *Hip on Health: Health Information for Caregivers and Families* by Charlotte M. Hendricks. Published by Redleaf Press. www.redleafpress.org.

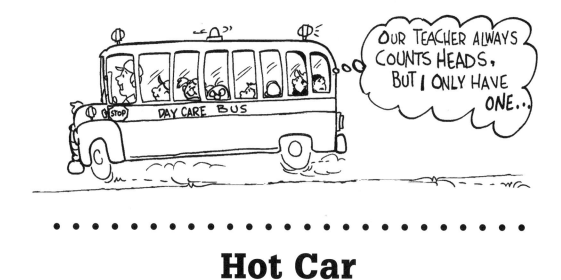

Hot Car

Never leave children alone in a car—not even for a minute. Every year, children suffer heatstroke from being trapped in vehicles, sometimes with fatal results. On a warm or sunny day, the temperature inside a vehicle can reach 120°F or higher in just a few minutes, even with the windows open. Check the back seat! A child left in a hot car can suffer serious injury or death in less than an hour.

How does this happen? A busy or exhausted parent going to work may not think about the child sleeping in the back seat. A caregiver transporting children may not check every seat before leaving the van.

Set up reminders to prevent this from happening:

✓ Put something you need, such as your cell phone, handbag, or your left shoe, in the backseat with your child.

✓ Tell child caregivers you will always call if your child will not attend. If your child is not dropped off at the normal time, they should call you within ten to fifteen minutes.

✓ Ask child caregivers how often they "count heads" when transporting children.

Children playing may crawl inside a car. If the door closes, they may not know how to get out. Help prevent these situations by locking the doors when you exit a vehicle.

Show children how to unlock vehicle doors, including electric locks, pull locks, and levers. A front door may open when a back door will not. Tell them to blow the vehicle horn for help. Also, show children how to use emergency escape latches in a car trunk.

If you see a child alone in a car, call 911 immediately!

From *Hip on Health: Health Information for Caregivers and Families* by Charlotte M. Hendricks. Published by Redleaf Press. www.redleafpress.org.

Insect Bites and Stings

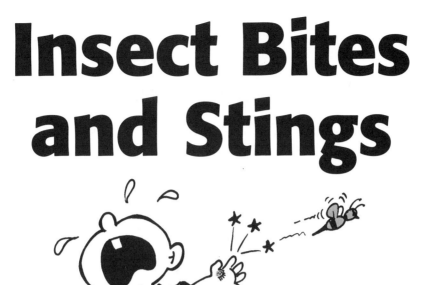

Bites or stings from ants, bees, or wasps can be dangerous if children are allergic to them. Many stings or bites at one time can also be dangerous.

Watch for these symptoms:

- problems with breathing or wheezing

- fainting

- hives or skin rash

- swelling of the face, mouth, or eyelids

From *Hip on Health: Health Information for Caregivers and Families* by Charlotte M. Hendricks. Published by Redleaf Press. www.redleafpress.org.

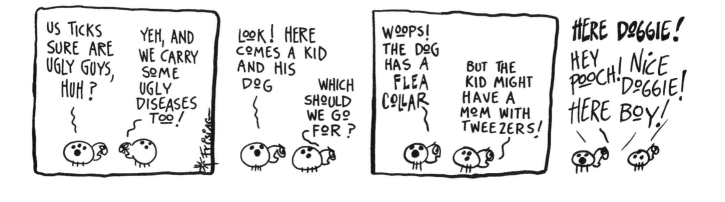

Insect Bites and Stings

Bug bites and stings can be a real nuisance, but most are not serious.

Mosquitoes, red bugs (chiggers), and fleas cause itching. If children scratch at such bites, they can develop skin infections. One way to stop the itch is to put a paste of baking soda and water on the bite. You also can ask a pharmacist about medicines for bug bites.

Bites or stings can be dangerous if children are allergic to them or if they receive many bites or stings at one time. If children exhibit swelling or breathing problems, call emergency help (911)!

Most spiders are not dangerous. Two poisonous spiders are the black widow and the brown recluse (fiddler) spider.

Ticks live in grass, weeds, trees, and on animals. Check children's skin and scalp for ticks. Ticks bury their heads into the skin when they bite. When children have embedded ticks, remove the ticks as soon as possible. The longer they stay on the skin, the harder they are to remove. Hold the tick with tweezers close to the skin. Pull slowly and gently to remove the tick.

Ticks can carry life-threatening diseases such as Lyme disease and Rocky Mountain spotted fever. When children have hosted embedded ticks, call their doctor immediately if they exhibit any of these symptoms:

✓ fever, chills, or headache

✓ rash or ring-shaped red spot that grows larger each day

✓ rash on hands and feet that spreads over the body

✓ stiff neck

✓ pain or swelling in the joints

From *Hip on Health: Health Information for Caregivers and Families* by Charlotte M. Hendricks. Published by Redleaf Press. www.redleafpress.org.

Insect Repellent

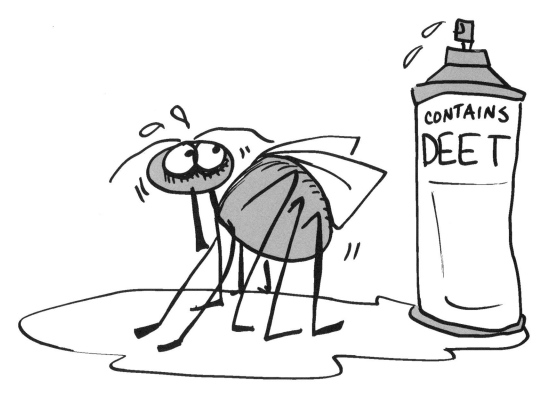

Try to prevent insect bites. Many insects carry disease.

Most insect repellents contain a chemical known as DEET. Repellents containing 30 percent DEET (or less) are safe for most children. Follow the directions on the label.

Do not use DEET products on infants younger than 2 months old.

From *Hip on Health: Health Information for Caregivers and Families* by Charlotte M. Hendricks. Published by Redleaf Press. www.redleafpress.org.

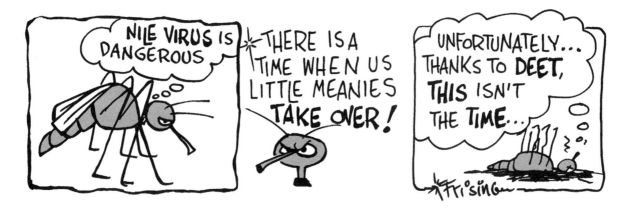

Insect Repellent

Many insects carry disease. For example, mosquitoes may spread West Nile virus, and ticks may carry Lyme disease and Rocky Mountain spotted fever. Try to prevent insect bites.

When outside, children should wear protective clothing as much as possible, including long sleeves and pants. If their clothes are thin, spray the clothes with insect repellent for extra protection. Most insect repellents contain a chemical known as DEET.

Not all repellents have the same concentration of DEET. The American Academy of Pediatrics recommends that products for children contain no more than 30 percent DEET. Follow the directions on the label. Protection can last several hours, depending on the product used.

Do not spray around children's faces. Instead, spray some repellent on your hands and rub it on children's faces, avoiding the eye areas. Do not put repellent on children's hands because they may rub their eyes.

Do not use DEET on infants younger than two months. Protect infants by placing mosquito netting over their carriers when they are outside.

The Centers for Disease Control and Prevention does not recommend products that combine sunscreen and DEET. Recommendations for safe use of sunscreen and safe use of DEET are different.

Lawn Mower Safety

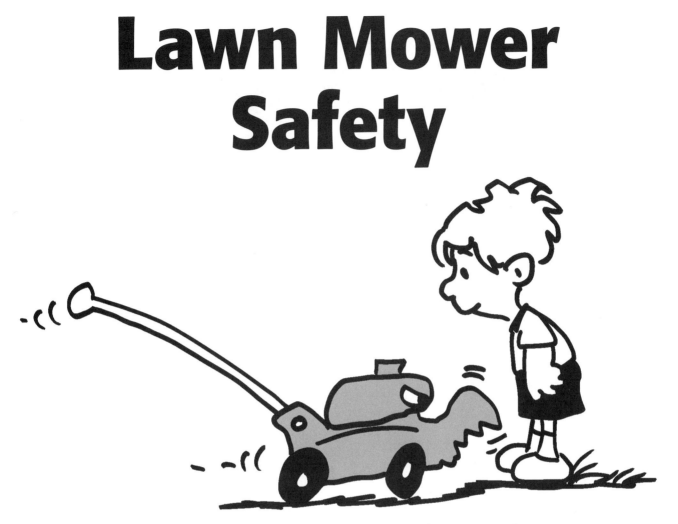

Most children are not tall or strong enough to use lawn mowers until about 14 years of age.

Riding mowers are not toys! Keep children off them. Children can fall under these blades.

Do not let children play nearby while you are mowing. Mowers can throw objects with great force and for long distances. Thrown objects can severely injure or kill a child.

From *Hip on Health: Health Information for Caregivers and Families* by Charlotte M. Hendricks. Published by Redleaf Press. www.redleafpress.org.

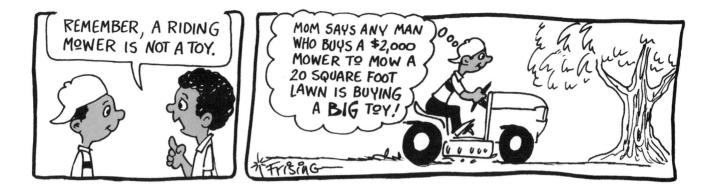

Lawn Mower Safety

Keep children away when using lawn mowers, weed eaters, and power tools.

Lawn mowers can throw sticks, rocks, broken glass, and other objects with great force and very far. If an object hits a child, it could cause serious injury or death. Weed eaters and blowers can also throw objects. Even small objects can injure a child's eye.

Most children are not tall or strong enough to use lawn mowers until about fourteen years of age. Once they are big enough, teach them the safe way to mow grass.

Riding mowers are not toys! Keep children off riding mowers. They can fall under these blades.

Here are tips to keep everyone safe:

✓ Wear goggles when using a weed eater and other power tools.

✓ Do not let children ride on mowers.

✓ Keep children away from the area when using mowers or weed eaters.

From *Hip on Health: Health Information for Caregivers and Families* by Charlotte M. Hendricks. Published by Redleaf Press. www.redleafpress.org.

Pedestrian Safety

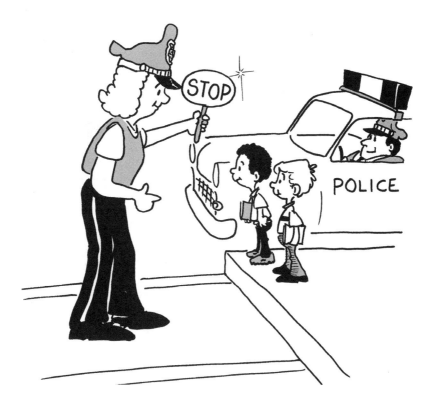

Children younger than 6 years old should not cross streets alone. The necessary "stop, look, and listen" skills are not fully developed before then.

Teach children the safe way to cross a street by being a good role model. Cross streets at the corner and wait until all traffic is past before stepping into the street.

Teach children to never go into the street after a ball or toy.

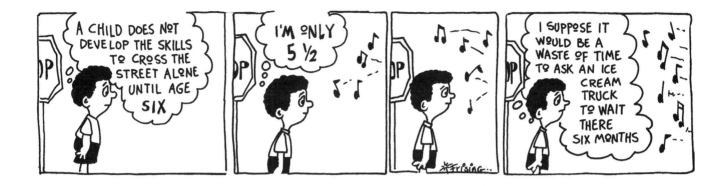

Pedestrian Safety

Children younger than six years old should not cross streets alone. Although some children seem to cross streets carefully, they do not always remember to stop, look both ways, and listen. The skills needed to safely cross streets do not develop until after age six.

Children make decisions based on what they can see, hear, and touch. They may believe that if they can see the car, then its driver will see them and will stop. Young children may hear the vehicle but cannot tell if it is coming closer or going away. Young children cannot judge distances or the speed of vehicles.

Teach children the safest way to cross a street. Model safe actions by crossing at the corner and waiting until the street is clear before stepping into the street.

Teach children these important safety rules:

✓ Always stop, look, and listen. Look right, then left, the right again before crossing.

✓ Cars and trucks cannot see you. You have to watch out for them.

✓ Never go into the street after a ball or toy. Toys can be replaced, but your body might get hurt.

✓ Stand away from the street while waiting to cross.

✓ Cross the street at the corner.

✓ Recognize "walk" and "don't walk" signs and traffic signals.

From *Hip on Health: Health Information for Caregivers and Families* by Charlotte M. Hendricks. Published by Redleaf Press. www.redleafpress.org.

Pet and Animal Safety

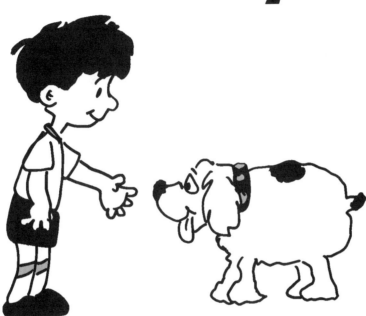

Help children learn to enjoy and respect animals.

Animals can be great friends.

Teach children to touch animals gently. They should not poke, pull, or hold animals too tightly. They should never tease or throw objects at animals.

Any animal, even their own pets, may bite if they hurt it. Animal bites or scratches can be serious, especially when children's faces are injured.

From Hip on Health: Health Information for Caregivers and Families by Charlotte M. Hendricks. Published by Redleaf Press. www.redleafpress.org.

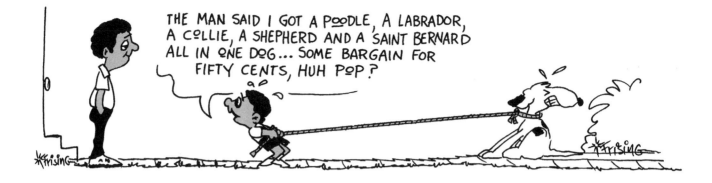

Pet and Animal Safety

Some children seem to have no fear of animals, while others are afraid. Help children learn to enjoy and respect animals. Animals can be great friends.

Animal bites or scratches can be serious, especially when children's faces are injured. Teach children to avoid stray animals or pets they do not know well. If they want to pet an animal and the owner says the animal will not bite, take the following precautions:

✓ Stay close to children to help prevent injury if an animal does jump, bite, or scratch.

✓ Let children hold out their hands and let the animal come to them.

✓ Do not allow children to pet animals that growl, lay back their ears, or act scared or aggressive.

Treat animals with respect. Touch gently and avoid poking, pulling, and holding them too tightly. Children should not tease or throw objects at animals. Any animal, even their own pets, may bite if they hurt it.

Pets can help children learn responsibility, but do not expect too much of young children. They can help with pet care, but adults should be sure the pet is cared for. Even older children do not always remember to feed, water, and care for their pets. Be sure pets have up-to-date shots, including rabies vaccine.

From *Hip on Health: Health Information for Caregivers and Families* by Charlotte M. Hendricks. Published by Redleaf Press. www.redleafpress.org.

Playground Safety

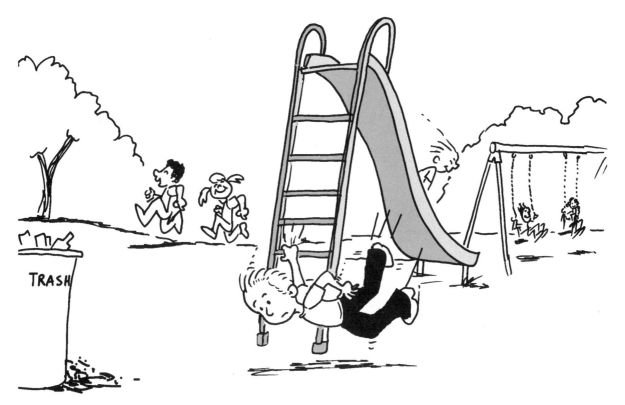

Playgrounds give children places to run, jump, and have fun being physically active. Adults must make sure that playgrounds are safe.

The greatest risk of injury is from falls. Play equipment should have soft surfaces under and around it, such as special playground surface material or deep sand or wood chips.

Check play equipment for sharp edges, nails, and broken pieces sticking out. Check the ground for pieces of glass and trash.

From *Hip on Health: Health Information for Caregivers and Families* by Charlotte M. Hendricks. Published by Redleaf Press. www.redleafpress.org.

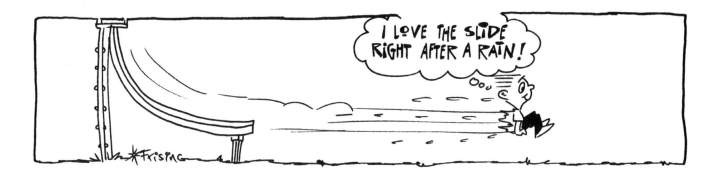

Playground Safety

Each year, about 200,000 children are treated at hospital emergency rooms for injuries occurring on playgrounds. Most injuries are caused by falls from slides, climbers, swings, or other equipment. Falls can cause serious injury or death.

Playground injuries are usually caused by one of four things:

✓ The equipment is too tall.

✓ The surfaces underneath equipment are hard.

✓ The equipment is broken or not anchored properly.

✓ Children are not properly supervised.

Falls onto hard surfaces, such as dirt, gravel, or concrete, can cause serious injury. Even grass is not safe for equipment more than three feet high. There should be a large area of special playground surface material or of deep sand, wood chips, or small pea gravel both under and at least six feet beyond all equipment. This softer surface helps prevent serious injury when children fall.

Parents and teachers should inspect play areas for equipment hazards, broken glass and debris, and wasp and fire ant nests. Children should always be supervised by a responsible adult and encouraged to follow safety rules to prevent injury.

From *Hip on Health: Health Information for Caregivers and Families* by Charlotte M. Hendricks. Published by Redleaf Press. www.redleafpress.org.

Prevent Head Injury

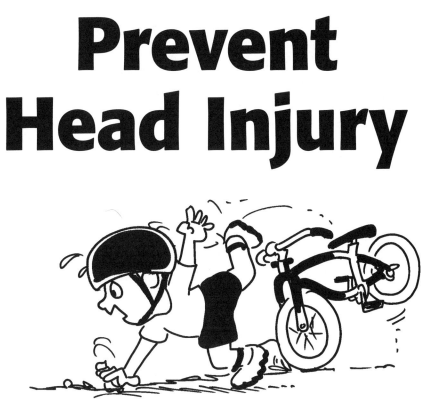

Falls can cause serious head and spinal injuries. When children fall or hit their heads, watch for signs of serious injury:

- bleeding from the nose, ears, or eyes

- fainting or unconsciousness

- dizziness, nausea, or vomiting

- dilated eyes

- numbness in arms or legs

If you notice any of these signs, call emergency help (911) immediately!

From *Hip on Health: Health Information for Caregivers and Families* by Charlotte M. Hendricks. Published by Redleaf Press. www.redleafpress.org.

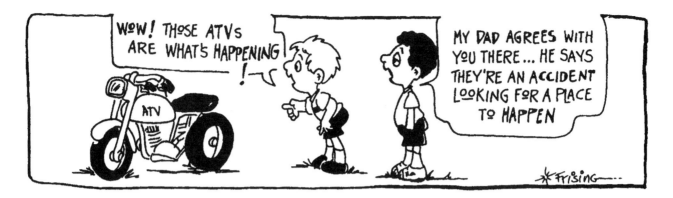

Prevent Head Injury

When children hurt their heads, necks, or backs, they may suffer from memory loss, loss of sight or hearing, brain damage, paralysis, or death. Brain and spinal cord injuries can cause permanent damage.

Common causes of injury in children are vehicle crashes, falling down steps or off playground equipment, and crashing while riding bicycles, motorcycles, or all-terrain vehicles (ATVs).

Here are some ways to prevent injury:

✓ Always buckle up with a safety seat or safety belt.

✓ Use safety gates at stairs. Do not allow children to play around steps.

✓ Watch children carefully on playground equipment. Do not let too many children play on equipment at one time. Young children should not play on tall equipment.

✓ Trampolines are dangerous, especially if more than one child uses them at a time.

✓ Teach children to wear helmets when riding bikes, in-line skating, or skateboarding.

✓ ATVs and motorcycles are not safe for children.

Check inside and around your home for objects that could fall on children. If they pull on a table, bookshelf, or concrete birdbath, the object could fall on them and cause serious injury.

From *Hip on Health: Health Information for Caregivers and Families* by Charlotte M. Hendricks. Published by Redleaf Press. www.redleafpress.org.

Sun Safety—Avoid Hot Surfaces

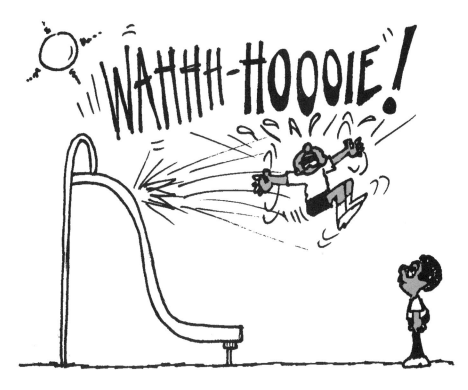

A child's skin is tender and can burn more quickly than an adult's skin. A child can get a serious burn from touching a hot surface, such as a playground slide, a safety seat, or a seat belt buckle.

Use the back of your hand to check for hot surfaces. If it feels warm to you, it will feel hot to a child's skin.

From *Hip on Health: Health Information for Caregivers and Families* by Charlotte M. Hendricks. Published by Redleaf Press. www.redleafpress.org.

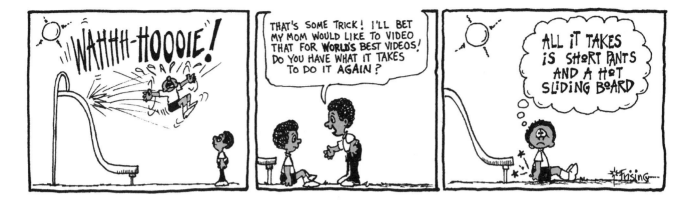

Sun Safety—
Avoid Hot Surfaces

The sun provides us with light and warmth, and is our primary source of vitamin D. But sunshine can make metal and other surfaces very hot. A child can get a serious burn by touching a hot surface, such as a playground slide or a car seat buckle.

A child's skin is tender and can burn more quickly than an adult's skin. Use the back of your hand to check for hot surfaces. If it feels warm to you, it will feel hot to a child's skin.

Here are some ways to avoid burns:

✓ Check the surfaces of slides and other playground equipment before children play on them.

✓ Place a towel over children's safety seats and seat belt buckles when you park the vehicle. When you return, check these items. If the buckle or seat is warm, turn on the air conditioner and cool the seat before buckling-up children. *Always use approved child safety seats and buckle up!*

✓ Be sure children wear shoes when playing or walking outdoors. Hot sidewalks, streets, and sand can burn tender feet.

Practice sun safety, every day, all year long.

From *Hip on Health: Health Information for Caregivers and Families* by Charlotte M. Hendricks. Published by Redleaf Press. www.redleafpress.org.

Sun Safety–Cover Up

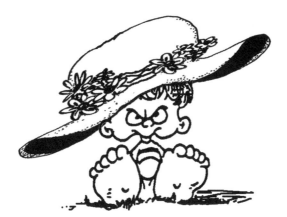

Clothing and hats help protect children from too much sun. Hats provide shade that you can take with you wherever you go!

Dress children in play clothes that are cool, comfortable, and cover most of their skin.

Practice sun safety, every day, all year long.

From *Hip on Health: Health Information for Caregivers and Families* by Charlotte M. Hendricks. Published by Redleaf Press. www.redleafpress.org.

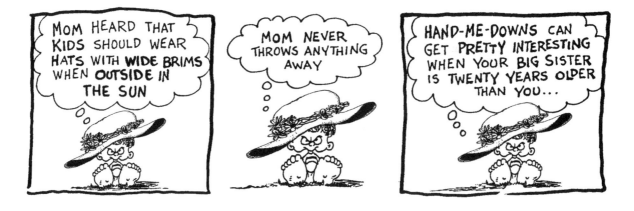

Sun Safety—Cover Up

Children need to play outside, but playing too long in the sun can lead to sunburn and skin damage. A sunburn can occur in just ten minutes during the midday sun even on cold days. Even children with dark skin can get skin damage. Research shows a definite link between sunburn, especially sunburns during childhood, and skin cancer.

Clothes and hats provide protection from the sun.

- ✓ Choose clothes that cover more skin. Long- and short-sleeved shirts provide more sun protection than tank tops. Capris and long pants protect better than shorts. Shoes and socks protect the feet and ankles.

- ✓ Dress with layers of clothing that can be removed to accommodate play and temperature changes.

- ✓ Light-colored clothing feels cooler because the fabric reflects heat. However, dark colors absorb the sun's harmful ultraviolet rays better and provide more skin protection.

- ✓ Tightly woven fabric provides more sun protection.

- ✓ Some companies offer "sun-safe" clothing that is light, durable, and ventilated. This clothing is labeled with a UPF (Ultraviolet Protection Factor) number to show its sun protective value.

- ✓ Hats with wide (four-inch) brims can shade the face, head, and neck. Safari-style hats with a flap in the back are the best.

Practice sun safety, every day, all year long.

From *Hip on Health: Health Information for Caregivers and Families* by Charlotte M. Hendricks. Published by Redleaf Press. www.redleafpress.org.

Sun Safety—
Infants

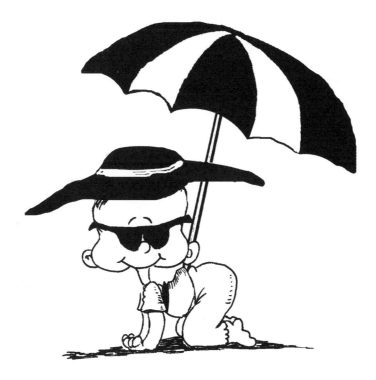

Keep your infant sun-safe.

Infants should not be exposed to direct sunlight. Stay in the shade.

Dress infants in loose-fitting clothing, including long sleeves and long pants.

Put a wide brimmed hat on infants.

From Hip on Health: Health Information for Caregivers and Families by Charlotte M. Hendricks. Published by Redleaf Press. www.redleafpress.org.

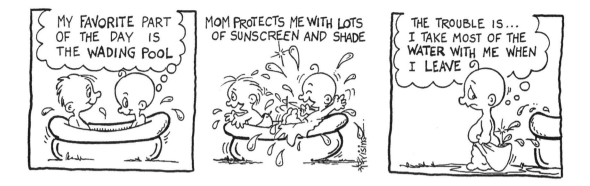

Sun Safety—Infants

Infants should not be exposed to direct sunlight. An infant's skin is delicate and can be easily sunburned in just a few minutes, even on a cloudy or cool day. Indirect sun rays reflected from sand, cement, water, snow, and ice can also cause sunburn.

✓ Keep infants in the shade.

✓ Cover infants with cool loose-fitting clothing. Do not overdress infants. Young children can easily overheat, leading to dehydration, fever, and life-threatening heatstroke.

✓ Protect infants' heads, faces, and eyes and with wide-brimmed hats.

✓ Protect eyes with lightweight sunglasses labeled "100% UV protection."

✓ Infants and young children should not ride in open top vehicles (convertibles). Apply window film to side windows for extra UV protection.

✓ If adequate clothing and shade are not available, then ask a doctor about using sunscreen on small areas of the infant's skin, such as the face or back of hands. Choose sunscreen products labeled "broad-spectrum" SPF 30 or higher. Choose products labeled "PABA-Free" and that contain titanium dioxide, avobenzone, or zinc oxide.

Plastic, vinyl, and metal surfaces on strollers, safety seats, and play equipment can get very hot in the sun. Check surfaces and buckles with the back of your hand. If it feels warm to you, then it can burn an infant's skin.

From *Hip on Health: Health Information for Caregivers and Families* by Charlotte M. Hendricks. Published by Redleaf Press. www.redleafpress.org.

Sun Safety–Stay in the Shade

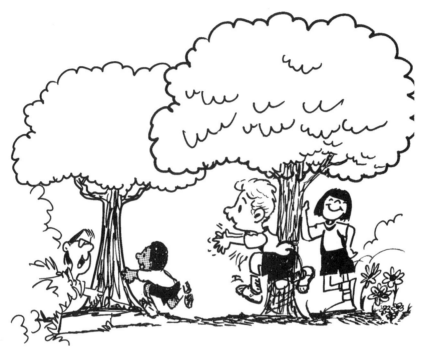

Stay in the shade during the sunniest part of the day. The sun is highest in the sky and has the strongest and most damaging rays from about 10:00 a.m. until 4:00 p.m.

Dense shade provided by large leafy trees, picnic shelters, awnings, and the shadow of a building keeps children cooler, and protects their skin and eyes from UV rays.

Practice sun safety, every day, all year long.

From *Hip on Health: Health Information for Caregivers and Families* by Charlotte M. Hendricks. Published by Redleaf Press. www.redleafpress.org.

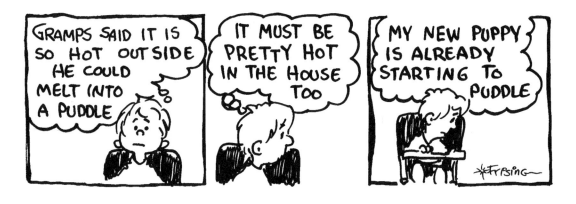

Sun Safety—Stay in the Shade

A big leafy tree provides welcome shade and makes playtime more fun on sunny days. Shade provided by trees, canopies, awnings, and the shadow of a building keeps children cooler, and protects their skin and eyes from UV rays.

Staying in the shade is most important during the sunniest part of the day. The sun is highest in the sky and has the strongest and most damaging rays from about 10:00 a.m. until 4:00 p.m.

✓ Look for dense shade; that is, solid shade with very few patches of sunlight. Buildings, picnic shelters, porches, and large leafy trees provide dense shade.

✓ Set up portable shade structures such as umbrellas, tents, and tarps.

If possible, build permanent shade structures such as porches, picnic shelters, or fabric shade canopies.

✓ Plan for the future by planting fast-growing broad-leafed trees in play areas.

Children also should be shaded from indirect sunlight. Sand and cement can reflect 10 percent of the sun's rays onto children. Water can reflect 20 percent, and snow and ice can reflect over 80 percent of UV rays! Look for large shady areas, preferably near grassy or other nonreflective areas.

The sun's rays can cause skin and eye damage even on cloudy or cool days. Practice sun safety, every day, all year long.

From *Hip on Health: Health Information for Caregivers and Families* by Charlotte M. Hendricks. Published by Redleaf Press. www.redleafpress.org.

Sun Safety– Sunburn

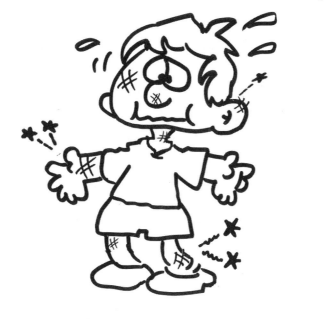

Children have tender skin. A short time in the sun can result in painful burns.

A single sunburn in childhood can increase a child's risk of developing skin cancer later in life.

There is no such thing as a healthy tan! Tanning, even from tanning beds, damages the skin and increases the risk of developing melanoma, the deadliest form of skin cancer.

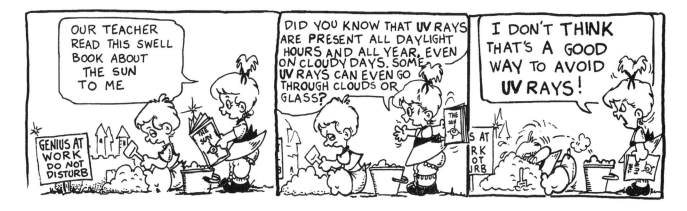

Sun Safety—Sunburn

Children need sunshine and outdoor play. Sunshine provides vitamin D, which helps their bodies absorb calcium for stronger, healthier bones. But too much sun exposure can cause sunburn.

Children have tender skin and a short time in the sun can cause painful burns. Even a single sunburn in childhood can increase a child's risk of developing skin cancer later in life. Some cancers, including melanoma, are life-threatening and can affect young adults.

If a child gets sunburned, the following tips may make him or her more comfortable:

✓ Have the child take a cool bath.

✓ Ask the child's doctor or pharmacist about remedies such as aloe vera gel or moisturizing cream. Avoid products with benzocaine or other ingredients which may cause additional skin irritation and pain. Do not apply products near the child's eyes.

✓ The child's doctor may also recommend an over-the-counter pain reliever like acetaminophen or ibuprofen. Do not give aspirin to children or teenagers.

✓ If the sunburn and pain is severe, if a child has a fever, or if blisters develop, call the child's doctor.

✓ Do not peel off loose skin. The skin underneath is at risk of infection.

✓ Keep the child out of the sun until the sunburn is healed.

There is no such thing as a healthy tan! Tanning, even from tanning beds, damages the skin and increases the risk of developing melanoma, the deadliest form of skin cancer.

Practice sun safety, every day, all year long.

From *Hip on Health: Health Information for Caregivers and Families* by Charlotte M. Hendricks. Published by Redleaf Press. www.redleafpress.org.

Sun Safety— Sunglasses

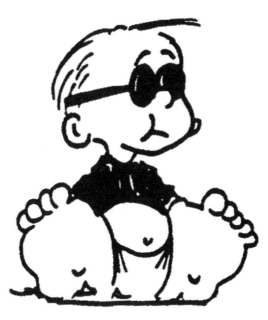

Sunglasses help protect eyes from the damaging rays of the sun. Choose sunglasses that are

- labeled "100% UV protection"

- have plastic or polycarbonate lenses that are impact resistant

- are lightweight and fit the child's face properly

Help children select sunglasses that they think are cool!

From *Hip on Health: Health Information for Caregivers and Families* by Charlotte M. Hendricks. Published by Redleaf Press. www.redleafpress.org.

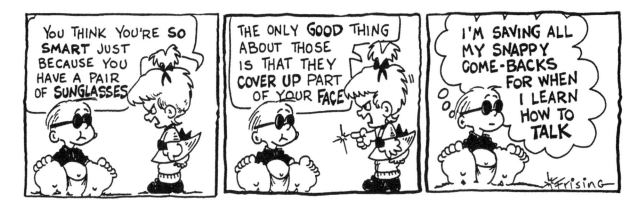

Sun Safety—Sunglasses

The sun produces ultraviolet (UV) rays that can damage the eyes. These rays are particularly damaging for infants and children under age ten because their eyes are more sensitive. Overexposure can increase the chances of developing eye disease.

Teach children to avoid looking at the sun and other bright lights. Wearing sunglasses is another way to help protect the eyes.

✓ Choose sunglasses labeled "100% UV protection" to protect against both UVA and UVB rays.

✓ If a child wears prescription eyeglasses, ask the eye care professional if the lenses have UV protective coating. If not, then ask for UV protective clip-on sun lenses.

✓ The color or darkness of the lens does not affect UV protection. Help a child choose sunglasses in a color and darkness that he likes, but you should also look through the lenses before buying them. Some colors affect the way the eye sees colors, brightness, and contrast.

✓ Choose plastic or polycarbonate lenses that are lightweight, impact resistant, and include UV protection.

✓ Select sunglasses that are lightweight and fit the child's face properly. Toddlers may want sunglasses in bright colors or animal shapes. Older children may prefer sunglasses similar to adult styles—sophisticated and trendy.

✓ Frames should be strong and durable. If the child is very active or plays sports, consider purchasing sports goggles, which also help protect the child's eyes from injuries.

From *Hip on Health: Health Information for Caregivers and Families* by Charlotte M. Hendricks. Published by Redleaf Press. www.redleafpress.org.

Sun Safety—Use Sunscreen

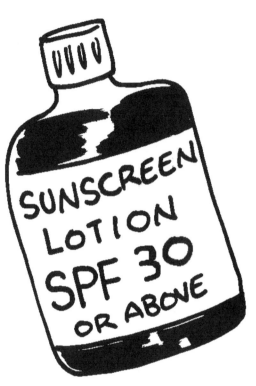

Too much sun can cause sunburn and damage skin. Children can get sunburn even on cloudy or cool days.

Protect children's skin by applying a sunscreen labeled SPF 30 or higher to all bare skin. Apply sunscreen about 20 minutes before going outside.

Reapply sunscreen every two hours if the child is playing outside.

From *Hip on Health: Health Information for Caregivers and Families* by Charlotte M. Hendricks. Published by Redleaf Press. www.redleafpress.org.

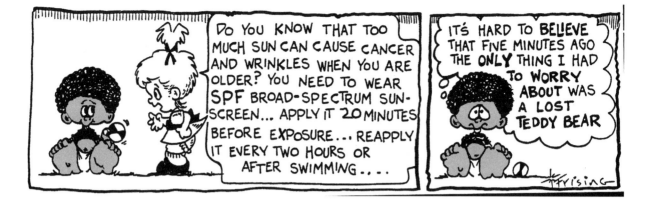

Sun Safety—Use Sunscreen

The sun's rays provide warmth and light, and children need outdoor playtime every day. But too much sun can cause sunburn or skin damage, even on cloudy or cool days. Hats, cover-up clothing, and seeking shade are the best ways to avoid overexposure.

Skin that is exposed should be protected with sunscreen.

✓ Choose sunscreen product labeled SPF 30 or higher. The SPF (Sun Protection Factor) is a scale for rating the level of sunburn protection. The higher the SPF, the more sunburn protection it provides.

✓ "Broad-spectrum" sunscreen provides protection from both ultraviolet A (UVA) and ultraviolet B (UVB) rays.

✓ Avoid combination sunscreen and insect repellent products because sunscreen should be reapplied more often than insect repellent.

Follow instructions on the product container.

✓ Apply sunscreen to all bare skin, including the ears and top of the head where the hair parts.

✓ Keep sunscreen out of eyes.

✓ Apply sunscreen about twenty minutes before the child goes outdoors.

Sunscreen products do not provide all-day protection. Generally, protection lasts about two hours. If the child will be playing outside longer than two hours, or if he is going back outside after two hours, apply more sunscreen. Also, reapply sunscreen after sweating a lot, playing in water, or toweling off.

From *Hip on Health: Health Information for Caregivers and Families* by Charlotte M. Hendricks. Published by Redleaf Press. www.redleafpress.org.

Water Safety

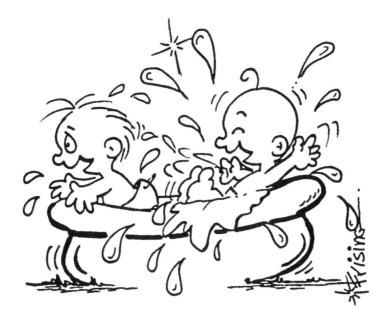

Children can drown in shallow water. Infants and toddlers can drown in just 1 or 2 inches of water because they do not know how to get out of it. Small children investigating a mop bucket or toilet can fall in headfirst and be unable to get out.

Never let children play alone around pools, lakes, or other bodies of water.

Swimming lessons are great for young children. However, this does not mean they can't drown.

From *Hip on Health: Health Information for Caregivers and Families* by Charlotte M. Hendricks. Published by Redleaf Press. www.redleafpress.org.

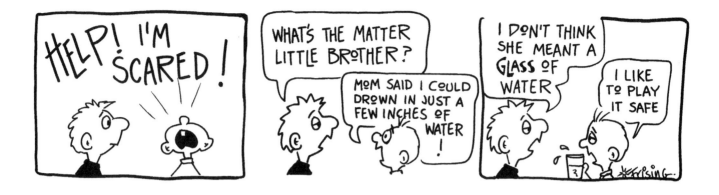

Water Safety

Never leave children alone in bathtubs, wading pools, or near water. Young children can drown in just a few inches of water. Infants and toddlers can drown in just one or two inches of water. If they fall headfirst into a mop bucket or toilet, they may not be able to get out and can drown.

Always watch children around pools, lakes, and other water. Even older children who know how to swim can get hurt or scared and may panic in the water. You should stay close in case children need help.

Water wings and floats will not keep a child from drowning. Children and adults in boats and watercraft should wear Coast Guard–approved life jackets or personal flotation devices.

Swimming lessons are great for young children. However, this does not mean they can't drown.

If children are diving into water, make sure the water is at least eight feet deep so they will not hit their heads on the bottom. Check first for submerged objects, such as rocks, tree stumps, or the steps in a pool.

Here are some water rules to follow:

✓ No running or pushing around the pool or water.

✓ Only one person on the diving board at a time.

✓ Never swim alone.

✓ Feet first to check the water depth. Only dive into deep water.

✓ Do not jump in on top of another person.

✓ Do not hold another child under water.

Weather Safety

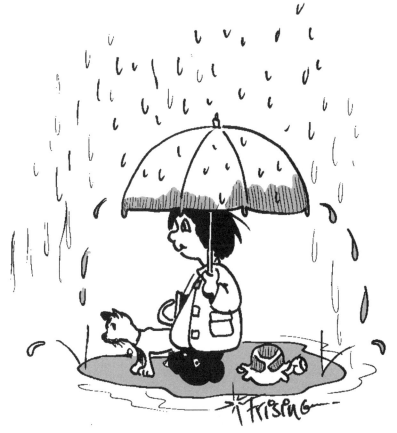

Playing in the rain can be fun. But often rain is accompanied by potentially dangerous weather conditions.

Lightning can strike anywhere. Children can be injured even in their own backyards. If you hear thunder, take children inside a building where they can safely enjoy the thunder-booms and light show!

Children learn by watching you. Always practice weather safety.

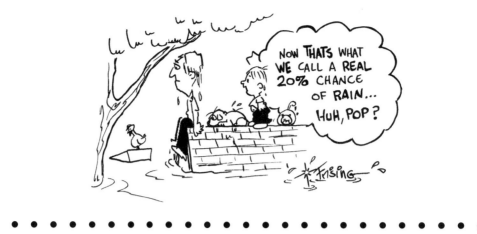

Weather Safety

There is truth in the old saying about "having enough sense to come in out of the rain." Getting wet does not hurt most children. But often rain is accompanied by potentially dangerous weather conditions.

If you hear thunder, take children inside a building where they can safely enjoy the thunder-booms and light show. Thunder and lightning go together, and lightning can strike anywhere. Children can be injured while on playgrounds or ball fields, in swimming pools, or in their own backyards.

When a lot of rain falls very fast, it can cause flash flooding. Water can run in dangerous currents through creeks and rivers, ditches, and down streets. Never allow children to walk or be driven through water, even if it looks safe.

Tornadoes can occur with little or no warning during thunderstorms or by hurricanes miles away. If large hail begins to fall during a thunderstorm, there may be a tornado nearby.

If a tornado warning sounds, such as a NOAA weather radio, a community siren, or smartphone alert, take children immediately to a safe shelter. The safest place is a small room on the lowest floor, away from windows, and near the center of the building. If you cannot get them inside a safe building, then make them lie down in a ditch or low-lying area. Have them protect their heads and faces with their arms.

Children learn by watching you. Keep calm and stay safe. Always practice weather safety.

Abuse and Neglect

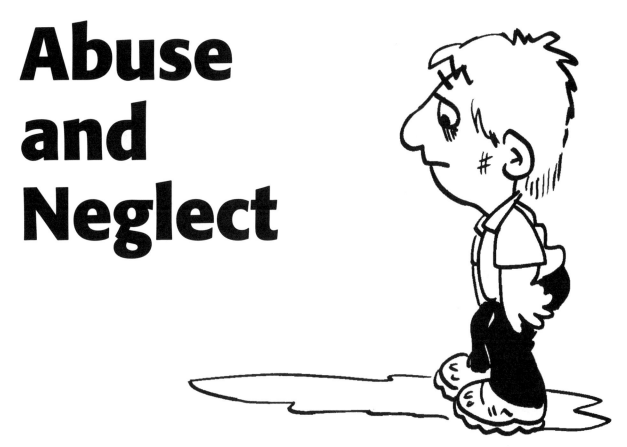

Abuse is physical, emotional, or sexual harm to a child. Some signs of abuse include the following:

- unexplained bruises or cuts

- burns from a cigarette, an iron, or from scalding

- pain, itching, swelling, or discharge in the genital area (private parts)

If you think a child is abused, call your local police department, health department, or children's hospital. The call will remain confidential.

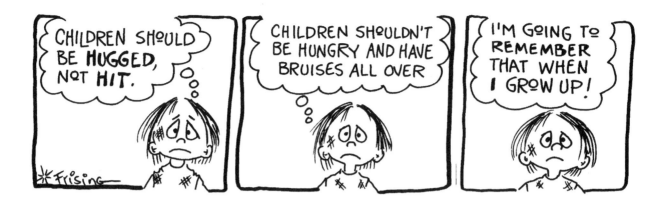

Abuse and Neglect

Childhood should be a happy time, full of love and affection, with enough food, clothing, and a safe place to live. Children need lots of hugs, smiles, and encouragement. Words like "I like the picture you drew" or "I love you very much" help children feel good about themselves.

Unfortunately, some children do not have safe and happy homes. Other children may be unsafe while in the care of individuals other than their parents.

Neglect is failing to provide for a child's normal needs, including food, shelter, and clothing. Some signs of neglect include the following:

✓ underweight or always hungry, begging for food, or stealing food

✓ dirty clothing or inappropriate clothing for the weather

✓ neglected sores, cuts, or other medical needs

Abuse is physical, emotional, or sexual harm to a child. Here are some signs of abuse:

✓ unexplained bruises or cuts, especially on the face, back, bottom, or genitals (private parts)

✓ burns from a cigarette, an electric iron, or from scalding

✓ pain, itching, swelling, or discharge in the genital area (private parts)

✓ frequent injuries that the child cannot explain

If you think a child is neglected or abused, call your local police department, Department of Human Resources, health department, or children's hospital. The call will remain confidential.

From *Hip on Health: Health Information for Caregivers and Families* by Charlotte M. Hendricks. Published by Redleaf Press. www.redleafpress.org.

ADHD

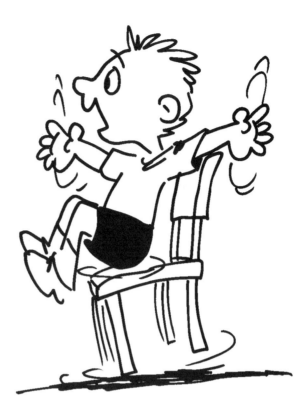

Children develop and learn at their own rates.

Most young children can sit still for three or four minutes when necessary. However, do not expect four-year-olds to sit still in chairs for ten minutes.

Some children have trouble concentrating. This medical condition is called Attention Deficit/Hyperactivity Disorder (ADHD).

Talk to the child's doctor if you believe a child has ADHD or other developmental problems, such as speech, hearing, or motor development (movement).

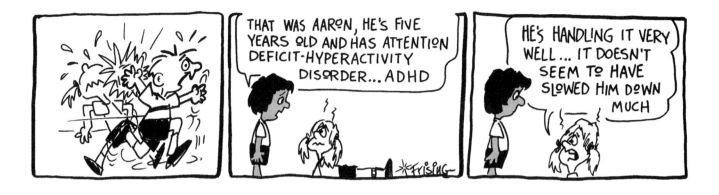

ADHD

Children grow and develop at different rates. One child may enjoy having you read aloud, while another child may not listen to even two pages. Some children sit quietly while others jump on their chairs. Most differences are a normal part of growing up.

Some children have trouble concentrating. This can make it difficult for them to pay attention and learn. This medical problem is called Attention Deficit/Hyperactivity Disorder (ADHD). Children with this disorder can have problems with their attention span, a high activity rate—always on the go (hyperactive)—and may act without thinking (impulsive). They may exhibit one or more of these behaviors. The cause of ADHD is not well understood.

All children go through stages when they may have one or more behavior problems. However, children with ADHD have constant behavior problems.

Talk to the child's teacher and doctor if you notice behavior problems regularly or if the child seems to have trouble concentrating and learning. Find out what the child is being asked to do and if it is age appropriate. For example, most young children can sit still for three or four minutes when necessary. However, do not expect four-year-olds to sit still in chairs for ten minutes.

Talk to the child's doctor if you believe a child has ADHD, or other developmental problems, such as speech, hearing, or motor development (movement).

From *Hip on Health: Health Information for Caregivers and Families* by Charlotte M. Hendricks. Published by Redleaf Press. www.redleafpress.org.

Biting

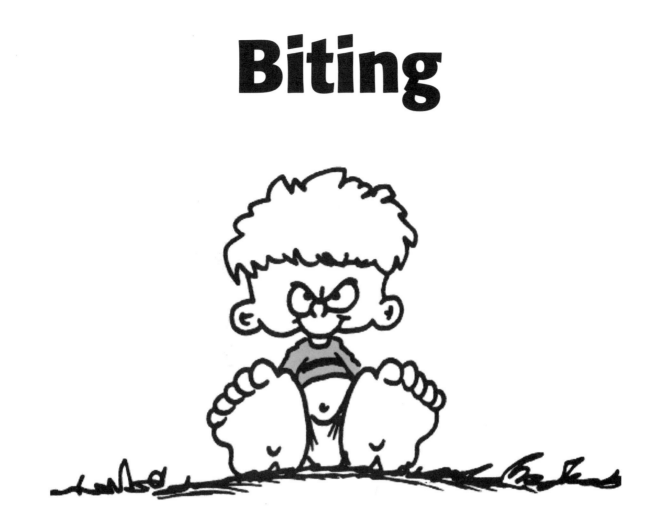

Many toddlers try biting. What can you do when they bite?

- Step in immediately between the child who bit and the bitten child.

- Look into the child's eyes and speak calmly but firmly. Say, "No biting people."

- Point out that biting hurts. Help and comfort the child who was bitten, and apply first aid.

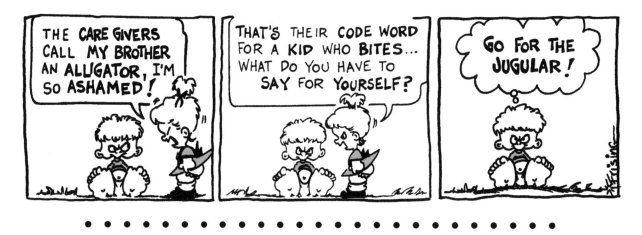

Biting

Infants and toddlers put their mouths on people and toys, and many toddlers try biting. Children bite for many different reasons. Some bite when they are mad or frustrated. Changes in their health or home life may cause biting. If you know why children are biting others, it will be easier to prevent the biting.

Watch to see when and where biting happens. Who is involved? What was the situation? What happened before and after the biting? Look for a pattern to the situations, places, or children involved. Can you see frustration developing in children just before they bite?

What can you do when children bite?

- ✓ Step in between the children. Stay calm.

- ✓ Look into the eyes of the child who bit and say calmly but firmly, "No biting people."

- ✓ Point out that biting hurts. Encourage the child who was bitten to tell the child who bit, "You hurt me."

- ✓ Help and comfort the child who was bitten, and apply first aid. If the skin is broken, wash the wound with warm water and soap. Apply an ice pack or cool cloth to help prevent swelling.

- ✓ Encourage the child who bit to help the other child by applying an ice pack or giving a gentle touch or hug.

Families of both children should be informed. The bitten child should be examined by a doctor if the skin is broken or redness or swelling occurs.

From *Hip on Health: Health Information for Caregivers and Families* by Charlotte M. Hendricks. Published by Redleaf Press. www.redleafpress.org.

Discipline with Love

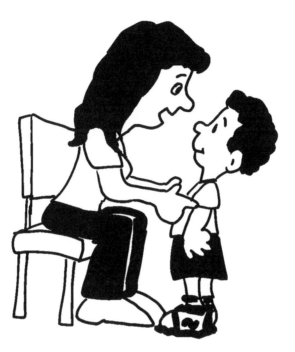

Never shake children, slap their faces, or hit their heads.

Children's brains are small and can move inside their skulls. If their heads are shaken or hit, their brains can bump against the skull and be injured.

This can cause vision or hearing loss, brain damage, or death.

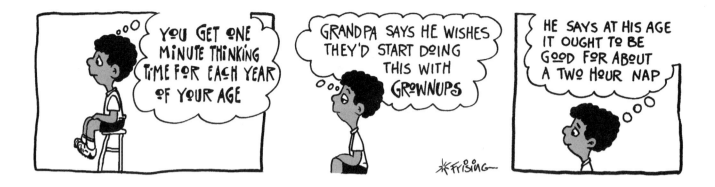

Discipline with Love

When you discipline children, let them know that their behavior is wrong, but that they are still good. Never tell them that they are bad. Instead, talk about their behavior.

Try to find out why they are misbehaving. Children may misbehave when they are sad, scared, tired, or sleepy. Help them learn to talk about what is bothering them.

All children go through stages when they act up. Some children bite, whine, and throw temper tantrums. Sometimes a four-year-old starts using baby talk again. Children go through times when they share their toys and times when they do not. Every stage is part of growing up. Help them learn appropriate behavior during each stage.

When you need to discipline children, try using redirection. This means to take them away from the situation and interest them in something else.

Another option may be time-out. Remove them from the situation and give them a few minutes to settle down and regain control of their emotions. Usually, an appropriate amount of time is one minute for every year of age. For example, a three-year-old might be in time-out for three minutes and a five-year-old might need five or six minutes to think.

Never shake, slap, or hit. A child's brain is small and can move inside the skull. If the head is shaken or hit, the brain can bump against the skull and be injured. This can cause vision or hearing loss, brain damage, or death.

From *Hip on Health: Health Information for Caregivers and Families* by Charlotte M. Hendricks. Published by Redleaf Press. www.redleafpress.org.

Effects of Alcohol and Drugs

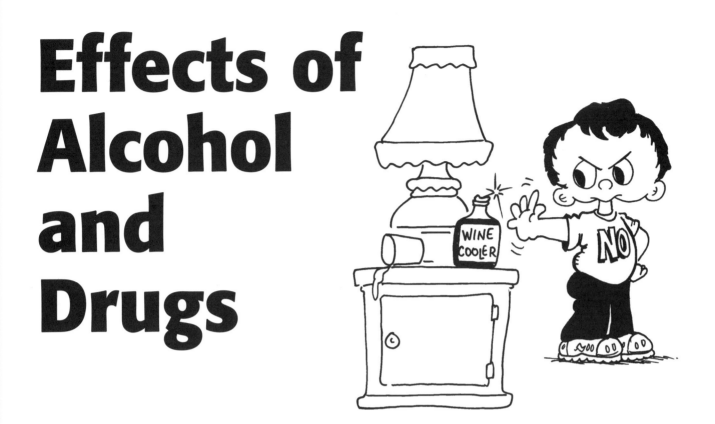

Alcohol is poisonous to young children! Even small amounts of beer, wine, and other alcoholic drinks can cause serious problems.

Alcohol lowers the body's blood sugar level. This can cause illness, coma, brain damage, or death. Do not let a child drink alcohol!

Many medicines and mouthwashes contain alcohol. Keep these out of children's sight and out of reach.

If a child swallows alcohol, call the Poison Control Center at 1-800-222-1222.

From *Hip on Health: Health Information for Caregivers and Families* by Charlotte M. Hendricks. Published by Redleaf Press. www.redleafpress.org.

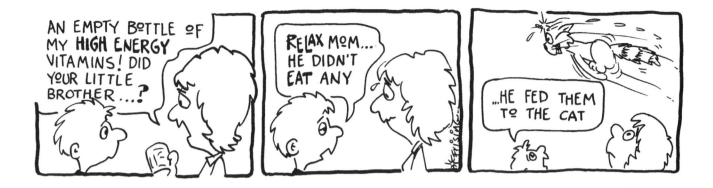

Effects of Alcohol and Drugs

The alcohol in beer, wine, cough syrup, mouthwash, and other substances can be dangerous for young children. Alcohol lowers the body's blood sugar and can cause illness, coma, or even death. Even a few sips of alcohol can cause serious problems for a young child. A single mixed drink could cause brain damage or kill an infant or toddler.

Do not leave beer and drinks where children can find them. Keep all alcoholic beverages, mouthwash, and cough syrup out of children's reach.

Children also can be poisoned by vitamins, sleeping pills, tranquilizers, blood pressure pills, and other medicines. Just one or two pills can cause problems ranging from upset stomachs to drowsiness, convulsions, coma, or death. Adult-strength iron pills are extremely poisonous for children.

Never call medicines *candy*. Teach children that medicine should be given to them only by certain adults. Tell them who is allowed to give them medicine—for example, parents, teachers, doctors, or nurses. *Tell them not to take medicines or drugs from anyone else!*

Always keep medicines in child-resistant containers. Store them in a locked cabinet out of children's sight and reach.

If a child swallows alcohol, medicine, or other substance, call the Poison Control Center at 1-800-222-1222.

From *Hip on Health: Health Information for Caregivers and Families* by Charlotte M. Hendricks. Published by Redleaf Press. www.redleafpress.org.

Effects of Caffeine

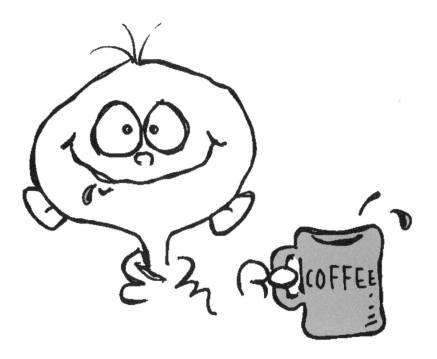

Pediatricians recommend that children avoid or limit caffeine use. Give children healthy, caffeine-free beverages such as water, 100-percent fruit juice, and milk.

Caffeine is found in many soft drinks, fruit-flavored beverages, coffee, tea, and chocolates. Read ingredient labels carefully on all beverages and look for "caffeine-free."

From *Hip on Health: Health Information for Caregivers and Families* by Charlotte M. Hendricks. Published by Redleaf Press. www.redleafpress.org.

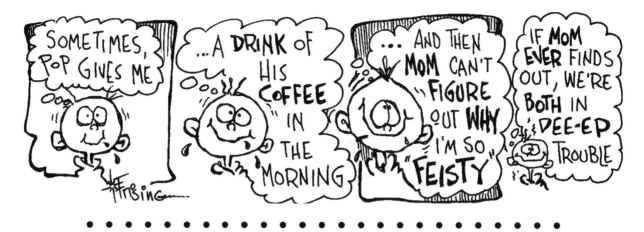

Effects of Caffeine

Do some children seem to be wired? Do they have trouble sleeping or resting at nap time? If so, the problem may be caffeine. Children who drink tea, chocolate milk, and soft drinks, or who eat chocolate candy, cookies, or cereal may be consuming caffeine.

Caffeine is a stimulant. When children consume it, their ability to perform tasks involving delicate muscular coordination, arithmetic skills, or accurate timing may decrease. Caffeine can also suppress children's appetites for nutrient-rich foods.

Caffeine takes several hours to leave the body. Consuming caffeine before nap time or bedtime may cause bed wetting or difficulty sleeping.

Pediatricians recommend that children avoid or limit caffeine. Give children healthy, caffeine-free beverages, such as water, 100-percent fruit juice, and milk.

Caffeine is found in many soft drinks, fruit-flavored beverages, coffee, tea, and chocolate items—including chocolate milk. Read the ingredient labels carefully on beverages and look for "caffeine-free." The term "decaffeinated" means that some, but not all, of the caffeine has been removed.

Teach children to avoid products with high levels of caffeine, including energy drinks. Too much caffeine can be harmful to children.

No Smoking!

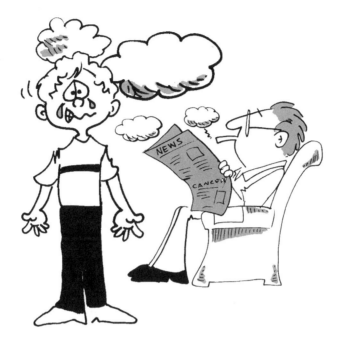

Smoke and residue from tobacco products can have harmful effects on everyone, especially children. Exposure to tobacco smoke and tobacco products can lead to asthma, sinus and ear infections, allergies, and respiratory problems.

Secondhand smoke is the smoke and other airborne products that come from burning tobacco products, such as cigarettes.

Thirdhand smoke consists of the smell, nicotine, and other chemicals left by tobacco smoke on skin, clothing, and other surfaces. To protect children, avoid smoking in your vehicle, home, and other places where children live and play.

From *Hip on Health: Health Information for Caregivers and Families* by Charlotte M. Hendricks. Published by Redleaf Press. www.redleafpress.org.

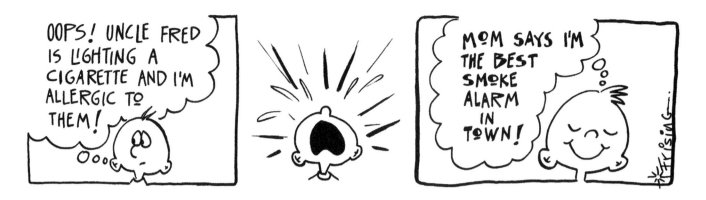

No Smoking!

Smoke and residue from tobacco products can have harmful effects on everyone, especially children. Exposure to tobacco smoke and tobacco products can lead to asthma, sinus and ear infections, allergies, and respiratory problems. Exposure to smoke increases the risk of Sudden Infant Death Syndrome (SIDS) in infants.

Secondhand smoke is the smoke and other airborne products that come from burning tobacco products, such as cigarettes.

Thirdhand smoke is the smell, nicotine, and other chemicals left by tobacco smoke on hair, skin, clothes, furniture, vehicles, and other surfaces. Thirdhand smoke remains long after smoking stops and is difficult to remove, even if you open windows or use fans.

Tobacco smoke is also harmful to unborn infants. If a pregnant woman smokes or is around tobacco smoke, her baby may not grow as much as it should during pregnancy. Infants who are born very small, or "low birth weight," often have more illness and physical problems.

Unfortunately, many children breathe cigarette smoke in their homes, restaurants, and stores. Teach children that smoking can hurt their bodies. Encourage children never to start smoking.

To protect them, avoid smoking in your vehicle, home, and other places where children live and play.

From *Hip on Health: Health Information for Caregivers and Families* by Charlotte M. Hendricks. Published by Redleaf Press. www.redleafpress.org.

Set Rules for Children

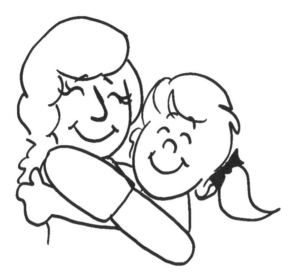

Children need lots of attention, love, and affection. Cuddling, hugging, rocking, and praise help them feel good and secure and helps their growth and brain development.

Another aid to children is to say "No" at the right time. Be consistent so they know what behavior is expected. Set reasonable rules and limits and stick to them.

Always let children know that you love them!

From *Hip on Health: Health Information for Caregivers and Families* by Charlotte M. Hendricks. Published by Redleaf Press. www.redleafpress.org.

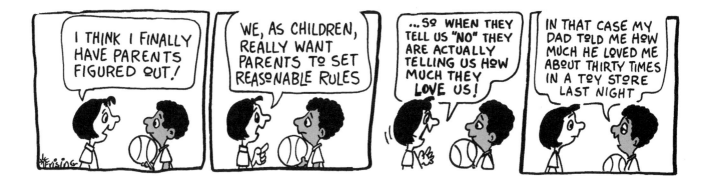

Set Rules for Children

Children need lots of attention, love, and affection. Cuddling, hugging, rocking, and praise help them feel good and secure and encourages their growth and brain development. Children also need consistent rules and expectations from adults.

Adults do not always know what they should expect from children. For example, at what age should you expect them to sit still, and for how long? Most young children cannot sit still for more than a few minutes. All children are different and develop at their own pace.

Parents and teachers can work together to understand what appropriate behavior to expect from children. Together, you can set limits and rules that are reasonable for their age.

Learn to say "No" at the right time. Be consistent—set reasonable rules and limits and stick to them. Children need to know what is expected of them.

State expectations in a positive manner. Tell children what you want them to do, rather than what they should not do. For example, tell children to "use quiet voices when indoors" rather than saying "Do not yell."

Always let them know that you love them. Everyone needs love and attention!

From *Hip on Health: Health Information for Caregivers and Families* by Charlotte M. Hendricks. Published by Redleaf Press. www.redleafpress.org.

Talk with Children

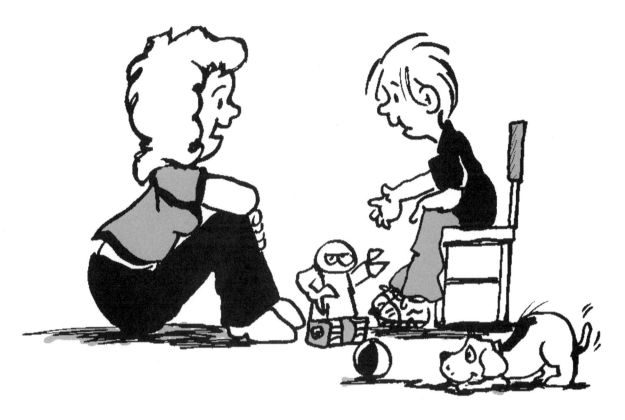

Build communication and trust by talking with children every day.

Listen to them. Show interest in what they have to say. Talk with children, not at them.

Encourage trust. If they tell you something that is just for you, then respect this confidence.

Answer questions honestly and simply.

From *Hip on Health: Health Information for Caregivers and Families* by Charlotte M. Hendricks. Published by Redleaf Press. www.redleafpress.org.

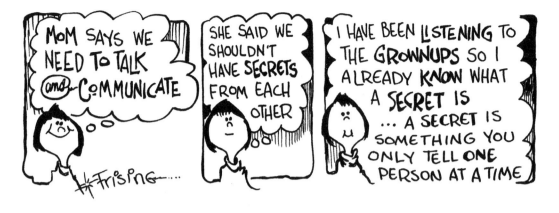

Talk with Children

Build communication with children during the early years. The benefits are enormous. Communication is essential not only to develop language skills but also for children's safety. Children who are lost in a store can tell someone their full name, your name, and their address. Toddlers who are injured can tell a doctor what part of their body hurts.

Build communication and trust by talking with children every day:

✓ Listen to children. Show interest in what they have to say. Turn off the TV and other distractions when they are talking. Spend one-on-one time with them every day.

✓ Talk with children, not at them. If they are learning a new skill or if you are correcting behavior, explain it in language they can understand.

✓ Encourage trust. If children tell you something that's just for you, then respect that confidence.

✓ Let children know that you are there for them. They should not be afraid to tell you something. Discourage secrets with other people.

✓ Answer questions honestly and simply. Do not laugh at children's questions.

The communication and trust built during childhood can continue throughout teenage years, but it requires work every day. The same technique—listening, showing interest, and building trust—also works with older children and teenagers. It even works with adults!

From *Hip on Health: Health Information for Caregivers and Families* by Charlotte M. Hendricks. Published by Redleaf Press. www.redleafpress.org.

Television and Children

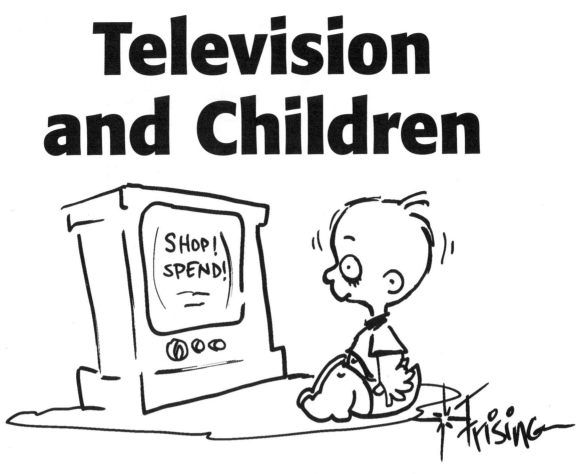

Children are constantly learning new things. The first three years of life are especially important for their brain development.

Too much exposure to electronic media (also called screen time) can negatively affect early brain development.

The American Academy of Pediatrics recommends avoiding television, DVDs, movies, video games, and games on computers, tablets, and phones for children two years or younger. Older children should not spend more than one or two hours per day on TV or computer/video games.

From *Hip on Health: Health Information for Caregivers and Families* by Charlotte M. Hendricks. Published by Redleaf Press. www.redleafpress.org.

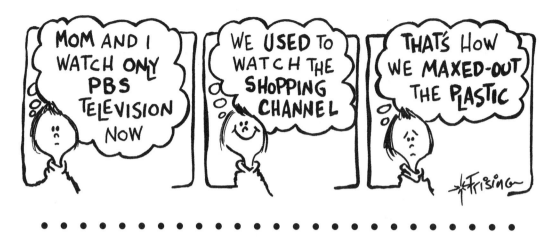

Television and Children

Children are constantly learning new things. The first three years of life are especially important to their brain development. Children need positive interaction with other children and adults while they learn to talk and play together. Screen time, including exposure to television, movies, computer games, tablets and phone games, even educational videos, are not as beneficial as interactions with real people.

Children who spend too much time in front of a screen do not spend as much time running, jumping, and playing. They are more likely to be less fit or overweight. They also may have poor sleep habits, poor focus, and more learning problems, especially in reading.

The American Academy of Pediatrics recommends that children two years or younger completely avoid television and other media. Older children should watch no more than one or two hours per day of high quality TV or computer/video games. When children want to watch TV or play screen games, consider the following:

✓ Choose educational programming, preferably with opportunities for children to copy activities like dancing or singing.

✓ Avoid programs and screen games containing violence.

✓ Watch programs and play games with children, then talk about them.

✓ Choose shows with limited commercials. Explain to children that commercials may make people want things they may not need.

From *Hip on Health: Health Information for Caregivers and Families* by Charlotte M. Hendricks. Published by Redleaf Press. www.redleafpress.org.

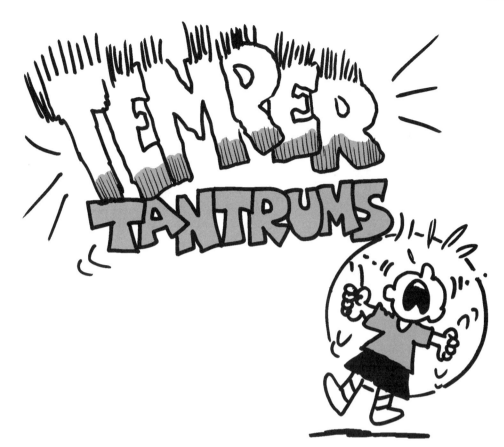

Toddlers sometime have temper tantrums. They are developing independence and think "I can do it myself" or "I want it—give it to me."

When toddlers discover that they cannot do something themselves or that they cannot have everything they want, they may throw tantrums.

Avoid putting children in situations that are likely to produce tantrums. Young children tire easily and have short attention spans. They should not be expected to sit quietly for long periods.

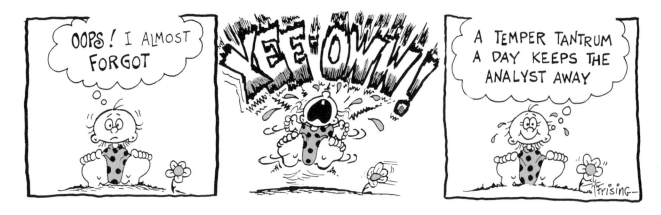

Temper Tantrums

Toddlers sometimes have temper tantrums. Some whine and cry; others may kick, hit, and hold their breath. Most tantrums are normal parts of children's development.

Tantrums usually occur when children become frustrated. Toddlers are developing independence and think "I can do it myself" or "I want it—give it to me." When they discover that they cannot do something themselves or that they cannot have everything they want, they may throw tantrums.

Avoid putting children in situations where tantrums are likely to occur. Young children have short attention spans and should not be expected to sit quietly for long periods. For example, they are likely to become bored or tired on shopping trips or in sit-down restaurants. They are more likely to throw tantrums when they are tired or hungry.

Do not give in to children during tantrums. Do not shake, spank, or scream at them. Here are positive ways to deal with tantrums:

✓ Offer children something to play with. Distract them.

✓ Take children to a quiet place to calm down. They may need a nap or something to eat.

✓ Ignore the tantrum if safety is not a concern and you are not disturbing other people.

✓ Hold children gently but firmly. They do not like to be out of control. Reassure them by being calm and showing love.

✓ Talk or whisper very quietly to children who are having tantrums.

Allowing children to make choices when possible helps prevent tantrums. For example, let them choose shirts and pants to wear—even if they do not match.

From *Hip on Health: Health Information for Caregivers and Families* by Charlotte M. Hendricks. Published by Redleaf Press. www.redleafpress.org.